PARTNER
WORKOUTS

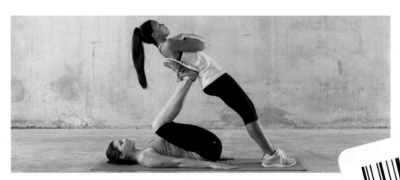

Team up and train with exerc[ises] you can do anywhere

Laura Williams
M.S.Ed., ACSM EP-C

CONTENTS

4 Stability Exercises

5 Programs & Workouts

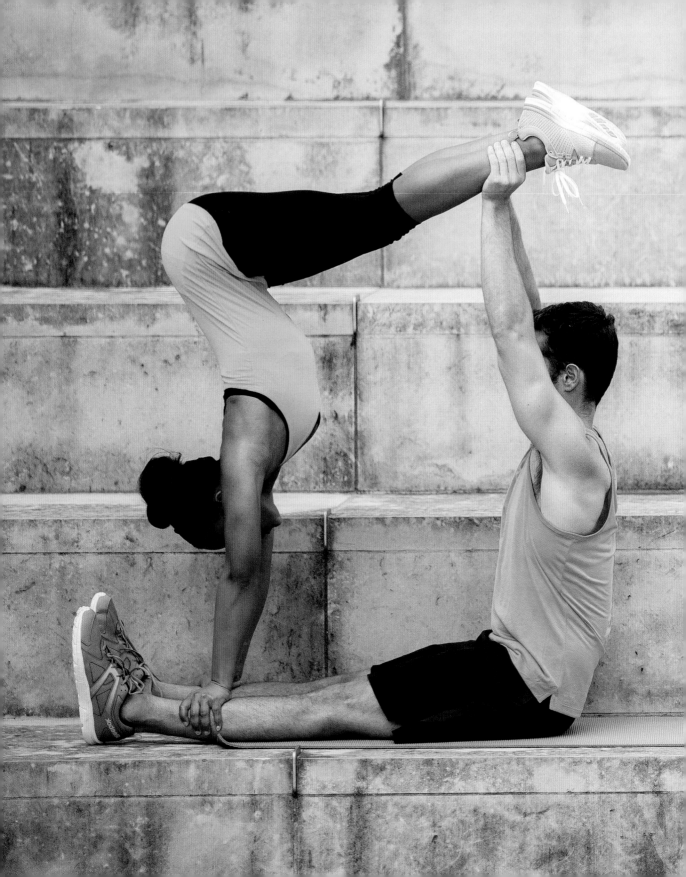

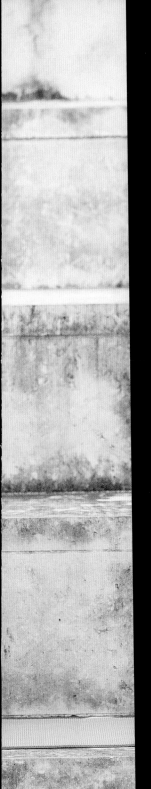

1

GETTING STARTED

Grab a friend (or a few!) and get ready for the best workouts of your life. This chapter teaches you the whys and hows of training with a partner, including proper form, warming up, and cooling down. Read this chapter carefully—it provides all you'll need to plan and execute perfect partner workouts.

INTRODUCTION

Partner workouts give you a chance to enhance and strengthen your exercise routines. They're more fun than exercising solo, and they offer a level of accountability: You're more likely to show up, get your sweat on, and see results when you've got a friend counting on you—and encouraging you. But the benefits don't stop there.

WHY WORK OUT WITH A PARTNER

FUN

Doing a million squats alone? Boring. Doing a million squats with a friend? An opportunity for laughter, bonding, and support. A workout buddy makes exercising feel more fun and easier—even when it's not.

PERFORMANCE

A 2012 study by researchers at Michigan State University found that people exercising with a partner worked out twice as long as those exercising alone—because they didn't want to be the first to stop.

CONFIDENCE

If you're ever unsure about how to properly perform an exercise, a workout partner can help reduce uncertainty and boost confidence as you become more aware of your own weaknesses.

MOTIVATION

Ongoing social support is one of the most effective means for starting and maintaining a fitness program. When you've got a friend encouraging you to work harder, you're more likely to actually work harder.

SAFETY

With a friend by your side, you'll always have someone there to help with balance, correct your form, and wave off shady characters, particularly if you typically exercise outside or in isolated locations.

RESISTANCE

Resistance exercises use an external source of resistance to enhance their movements. For example, to perform a resistance exercise, you might need a dumbbell, a resistance band, or a medicine ball—a requirement that will make that particular exercise more effective.

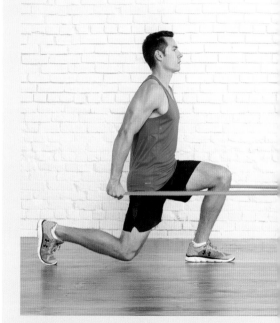

EXERCISE ORGANIZATION

Exercises in this book are categorized by three types—separated into chapters: resistance, assisted pairings, and stability. Some exercises fit more than one category. For example, an exercise using a BOSU ball might have a stability aspect but appears in the resistance or assisted pairings chapter because the primary intent of that exercise falls into one of these categories.

ASSISTED PAIRINGS

Assisted pairings exercises use your own or your partner's body weight as the primary source of resistance or challenge. An external source of resistance, like a dumbbell or a resistance band, isn't required, although using such equipment can make the movements harder.

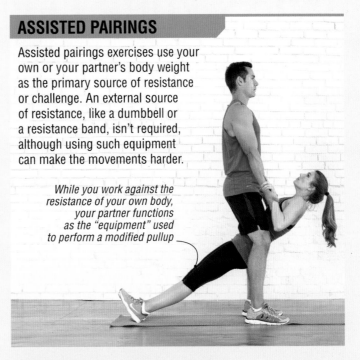

While you work against the resistance of your own body, your partner functions as the "equipment" used to perform a modified pullup

Resistance bands provide the external source of resistance required for doing triceps extensions

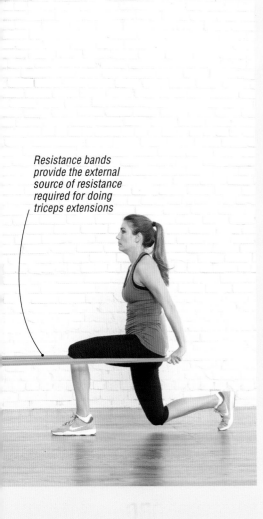

STABILITY

Stability exercises offer a neuromotor challenge, helping you develop balance, stability, coordination, and agility. Many of these also utilize equipment, but incorporating equipment is secondary to the neuromotor challenge.

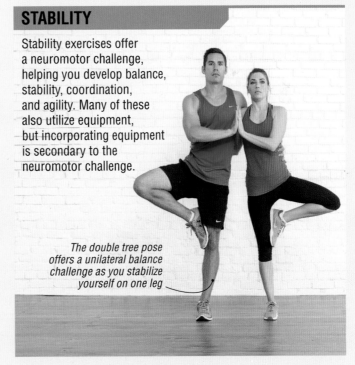

The double tree pose offers a unilateral balance challenge as you stabilize yourself on one leg

Along with the exercises being classified into specific categories, they're also separated into levels of difficulty. While these levels are a good indicator of a particular exercise's challenge, don't overlook exercises simply because they fall into a level outside your comfort zone. Many exercises include alternative versions that offer an easier or harder variation.

ASSESS YOUR LEVEL

If you don't know where you're starting, how will you know what you've achieved? Aside from helping you track your improvement over weeks or months, an initial fitness assessment can help you achieve your goals. After taking these tests, you'll know which level to start at in this book.

Write down your results so you can refer to them later. Retest your general fitness at periodic intervals to track your changes over time.

FITNESS TESTS

This simple personal fitness assessment enables you to determine your starting level for this book.

1
Perform all four tests in order without first warming up. Rest just long enough to recover between tests.

2
The test results will convert to a certain number of points. Turn the page and refer to the chart for your age group to find these points. Write them down.

3
Add up your points. Refer to the key below the charts to determine which level to start with.

TEST 1

3-MINUTE STEP TEST
Purpose Gauges your cardiovascular fitness based on your heart's ability to recover after exertion, as measured by your heart rate

Equipment 12-inch (31cm) step or bench, timer with a second hand, and metronome (or find a free metronome app)

1 Set the metronome to 96 beats per minute (bpm).

2 Stand with the step or bench in front of you. Step up one foot after the other, then down one foot after the next, moving in sync with the metronome, for 3 minutes. Alternate your lead foot each time you step up.

3 Sit down to count your heart rate for 1 minute using your carotid pulse (at your neck). Turn the page and refer to the chart for your age group to convert your heart rate to points.

TEST 2

1-MINUTE PUSHUP TEST
Purpose Assesses your upper-body muscular strength and endurance, as measured by how many reps you can perform

Equipment Timer

1 Men should assume a standard pushup position, supported by their hands and feet. Women should assume a modified pushup position, supported by their hands and knees.

2 Have your partner monitor your time, counting as you perform as many full pushups as possible in 1 minute. You should lower yourself to within 3 inches (7.5cm) of the floor before fully straightening your arms.

3 Turn the page and refer to the chart for your age group to convert the number of reps you performed into points.

WHY NOT FACTOR IN WEIGHT AND BMI?

Weight and BMI (body mass index) don't actually convey much information about internal health. It's possible to have a low BMI or weight while still having an unhealthy body composition. Likewise, it's possible to have a high BMI or weight while having a healthy body composition.

If weight loss is an important goal, you can monitor it in relation to measurements that provide more information about internal health, like tape measurements that track changes in body size at specific sites, particularly the belly (which is associated with heart disease), or body fat testing (which conveys more information about fat mass and lean mass), which is associated with overall health.

How you look and feel—are you energized and are you free of injury or illness?—are also good indicators of your overall health and wellness. If you feel the need to track your BMI or weight, don't lose sight of your other fitness goals.

TEST 3

1-MINUTE SQUAT TEST

Purpose Gauges your lower-body muscular strength and endurance, as measured by how many reps you can perform

Equipment Timer, sturdy chair

1 Stand in front of the chair.

2 Have your partner monitor your time, counting as you perform as many squats as possible in 1 minute. When you squat down, lightly touch your glutes to the chair (but don't sit all the way down) before returning to standing.

3 Turn the page and refer to the chart for your age group to convert the number of reps you performed into points.

TEST 4

1-MINUTE SITUP TEST

Purpose Assesses your abdominal and core muscular strength and endurance, as measured by how many reps you can perform

Equipment Timer

1 Lie on the floor, with your knees bent and your feet flat. Rest your hands lightly on your upper thighs.

2 Have your partner monitor your time, counting as you perform as many situps as possible in 1 minute. Use your abdominals to roll your torso to sitting as your hands slide up your thighs to your knees.

3 Turn the page and refer to the chart for your age group to convert the number of reps you performed into points.

HOW TO TAKE YOUR PULSE

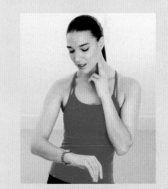

To take your pulse at your neck, place your index and middle fingers under your jaw on the side of your neck (at your carotid artery).

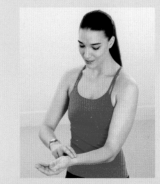

You can also take your pulse on either wrist by placing your index and middle fingers across your opposite wrist.

CONVERT YOUR POINTS

Refer to the chart for your age group to convert your test results from the previous pages into points. Add together all your points and refer to the key at the bottom of this page to determine your starting level in this book. Because each test's scores are adapted from standardized testing charts, you have some flexibility to move up or down a level as needed. When in doubt, start with an easier level and move up a level if the workouts and exercises feel too easy.

AGE 18–35

TEST 1	106–200 bpm	90–105 bpm	50–89 bpm
TEST 2	0–15 reps	16–35 reps	36+ reps
TEST 3	0–28 reps	29–39 reps	40+ reps
TEST 4	0–25 reps	26–43 reps	44+ reps
POINTS	1	2	3

AGE 36–55

TEST 1	110–180 bpm	95–109 bpm	50–94 bpm
TEST 2	0–10 reps	11–30 reps	31+ reps
TEST 3	0–23 reps	24–37 reps	38+ reps
TEST 4	0–20 reps	21–39 reps	40+ reps
POINTS	1	2	3

AGE 56–65

TEST 1	115–164 bpm	100–114 bpm	60–99 bpm
TEST 2	0–8 reps	9–24 reps	25+ reps
TEST 3	0–15 reps	16–29 reps	30+ reps
TEST 4	0–15 reps	16–30 reps	31+ reps
POINTS	1	2	3

AGE 66+

TEST 1	118–155 bpm	100–114 bpm	60–97 bpm
TEST 2	0–5 reps	6–23 reps	24+ reps
TEST 3	0–15 reps	16–27 reps	28+ reps
TEST 4	0–12 reps	13–29 reps	30+ reps
POINTS	1	2	3

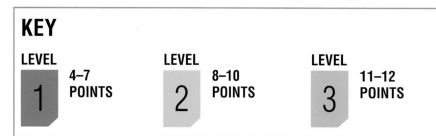

KEY

LEVEL 1 4–7 POINTS

LEVEL 2 8–10 POINTS

LEVEL 3 11–12 POINTS

You can repeat the Level 3 program as many times as you'd like. You can also make each exercise more difficult by increasing the resistance.

HOW TO USE THIS BOOK

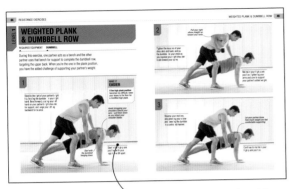

Each exercise has colored lines above the instructions that match the partners' shirts

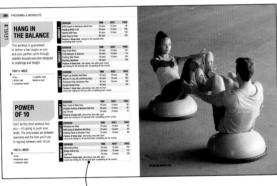

Each workout incorporates exercises from this book

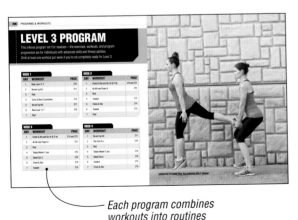

Each program combines workouts into routines

EXERCISES

This book provides 70 exercises divided into three levels of difficulty. Most exercises offer modifications to make the movements easier or more challenging. Although you'll perform the exercises as part of workouts and programs, you can also perform them on their own or as part of a workout or program you create.

WORKOUTS

Workouts are divided into three difficulty levels, and they consist primarily of exercises from their same level of difficulty. Workouts vary in format and length, offering a variety of sequences to keep your body guessing and progressing.

PROGRAMS

This book offers three 30-day workout programs, which are separated by difficulty level. After completing one program, you can repeat it additional times or progress to the next program. If you start using this book as a beginner, you can progress through this book at your pace, aiming to eventually complete the Level 3 workout program.

THE METHOD

1

Warm up before every workout by using the provided warmup exercises.

2

Based on your assessment, choose the workout suggested on Day 1 of the appropriate workout program.

3

Turn to the workout page and perform the exercises, accessing individual exercise pages as needed for further instruction.

4

Wrap up each workout with the provided cooldown stretches.

5

Continue following the workout program for 30 days. After a month, reassess your fitness level and either repeat the program or proceed to the next one.

CHOOSING A PARTNER

The exercises and workouts provided in this book require partners to actively engage with one another during each exercise. This sometimes means lifting your partner's weight or jumping over your partner's back. While selecting a partner has no hard and fast rules, you don't want to make the choice lightly.

HEIGHT

It's a good idea to select a partner within 4 inches (10cm) of your own height. When one partner is taller than the other, there's a corresponding difference in torso, leg, and arm length that can make many partner exercises more difficult.

WEIGHT

Find a partner within 20 to 30 pounds (9 to 14kg) of your body weight to set yourself up for greater success. Like height, weight differences between partners can make or break certain exercises. Picking a partner who is close to your weight will help during exercises where you have to lift or support each other.

FITNESS LEVEL

Try to choose a partner who has a similar fitness level. If you and your partner are at drastically different levels, one of you will constantly have to compromise your own workout to match your partner's level.

FITNESS GOALS

Partner with someone who wants to see gains in the same areas you do. For example, if your ultimate goal is to put on 30 pounds (14kg) of muscle mass but your partner wants to become more flexible, your goals might be at odds. It's best to work with someone whose goals are similar to your own.

WHEN YOUR PARTNER ISN'T THE PERFECT MATCH

It's absolutely okay to exercise with a partner of a different height, weight, or fitness level, but it may require some adjustments. Before tackling any of the provided workouts, test each exercise to make sure you both feel comfortable performing the movements as described. If you don't, find another exercise you both can do and substitute it into the workout. And don't feel like you have to have the same partner for all the workouts.

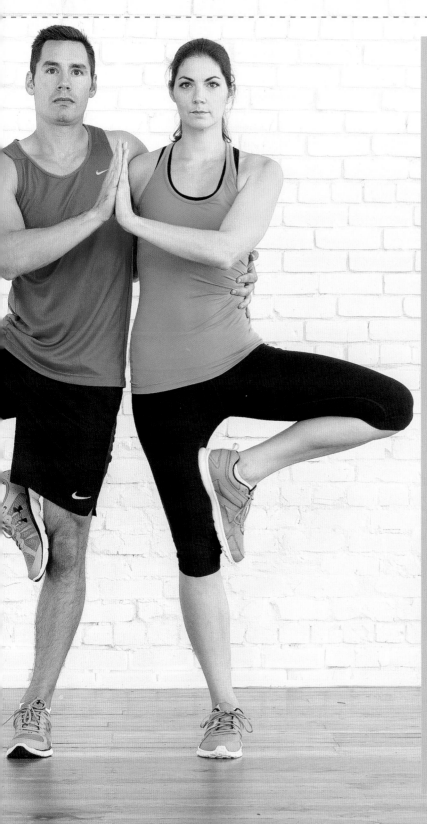

PLANNING YOUR WORKOUT

Choose a location

Partner workouts require more space than single routines because you're exercising with double the bodies. Choose spaces that offer room to move, like parks, aerobic centers, or basketball courts. Because many exercises require equipment, make sure you have access to what you need.

Opt for circuit training

Workouts in this book are primarily designed as circuits. This type of training keeps both partners moving to help elevate your heart rates for a greater cardiovascular challenge. Make sure you read each workout's instructions carefully so you understand how to cycle through the exercises, accounting for work and rest periods.

Select resistance and intensity

You don't need to always match your partner on resistance or intensity. This is particularly true when using medicine balls, dumbbells, and resistance bands. Feel free to select tools that vary in resistance from your partner. And when it comes to intensity, remember to go at your own pace. Workouts should feel challenging, not excruciating.

Set a few rules

It's not unusual for partners to have slightly different expectations about this experience. If you're looking forward to a hard session and your partner wants to chat the whole time, you're likely to feel frustrated. Talk with your partner about expectations, including how much notice to provide before canceling a workout and how much you want to talk while you exercise. Aligning expectations will improve the experience.

WHAT YOU'LL NEED

While many of the exercises in this book require no equipment, others incorporate balance and resistance tools to help you maximize each workout. By incorporating external equipment, you give yourself more options while providing the means to further improve your strength, balance, and coordination.

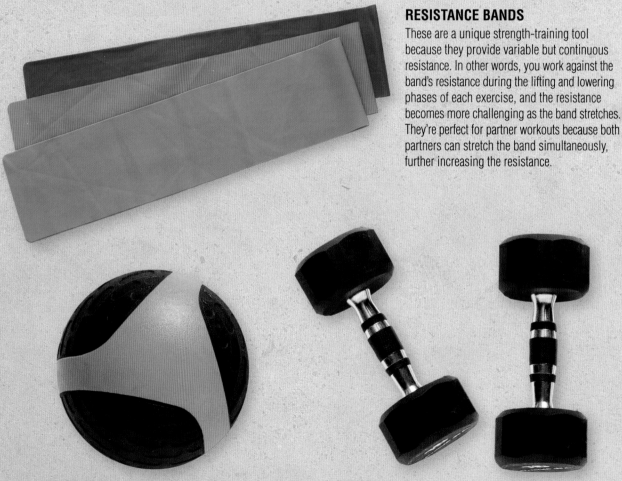

RESISTANCE BANDS

These are a unique strength-training tool because they provide variable but continuous resistance. In other words, you work against the band's resistance during the lifting and lowering phases of each exercise, and the resistance becomes more challenging as the band stretches. They're perfect for partner workouts because both partners can stretch the band simultaneously, further increasing the resistance.

MEDICINE BALL

It's hard to throw and catch a medicine ball when exercising alone, but with a partner, you can perform an array of exercises, including those that increase upper-body power and coordination, which are challenging to do alone.

DUMBBELLS

There's a reason dumbbells are a staple in gyms across the world: They're reliable and effective. Whenever you're looking to make an exercise harder, increase the weight of the dumbbells you're using or add dumbbells to the exercise.

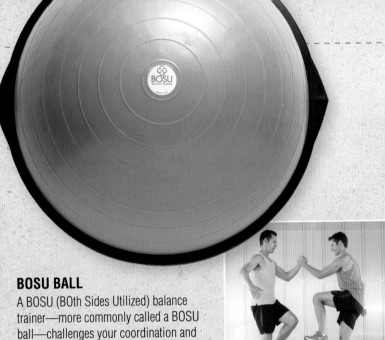

OTHER USEFUL EQUIPMENT

• **Timer:** Because most workouts are set up in a circuit or interval format, you'll need to track your work and rest periods. Download an interval timer on your phone or tablet so you can make adjustments to the timed intervals as needed.

• **Shoes:** A high-quality pair of athletic shoes will support you during your workouts and protect you from the elements. Don't buy shoes based on brand or price—buy them based on fit and comfort.

• **Water bottle:** Staying hydrated before, during, and after your workout is vital to your performance. Always carry a water bottle, and take a break every 10 to 15 minutes during a workout to drink several ounces. There's no need to spend money on sports drinks—basic water is best.

• **Yoga mat:** While yoga mats aren't a fundamental requirement for any specific exercise or workout, it's always good to have access to one. This is particularly true when one or both partners are sitting or lying on the floor.

BOSU BALL

A BOSU (BOth Sides Utilized) balance trainer—more commonly called a BOSU ball—challenges your coordination and balance, while its unique shape makes balance training more accessible. Use the BOSU ball dome side up for easier versions of stability exercises or flip it over for a greater challenge.

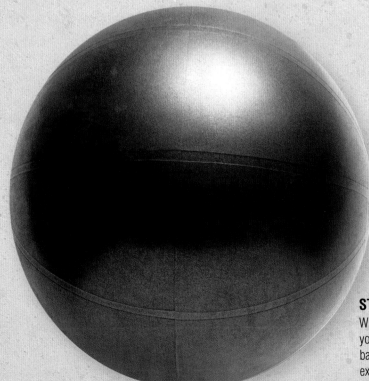

STABILITY BALL

When you add a stability ball or two to a partner workout, you add a new element of fun. You and your partner can balance, bump, and roll your way through a series of exercises you simply can't do on your own.

ANATOMY

These diagrams are designed to provide accessible and understandable descriptions of musculature. They offer a resource to better understand your body and how its different muscles are used during specific exercises to improve your strength, balance, and coordination.

Pectorals (Chest)
The three major muscles of the chest—the pectoralis major, pectoralis minor, and serratus anterior—all play a role in shoulder movement and stabilization.

Deltoids (Shoulders)
Consisting of anterior, posterior, and lateral muscles, the deltoids enable you to lift and rotate your arms.

Biceps
This "show me" muscle consists of two heads and helps with shoulder flexion, elbow extension, and hand rotation.

Abdominals
There's more to your abdominals than the rectus abdominis—commonly known as the *six-pack muscles*.

Rectus abdominis
This runs the length of your torso to help maintain posture and enables you to flex your spine.

Quadriceps
The quads consist of four major muscles: the rectus femoris, vastus lateralis, vastus medialis, and vastus intermedius. They enable you to bend your knee—a motion that's key in exercise and everyday movement.

Transverse abdominis
This deep muscle of your abdomen helps provide pelvic and spinal stability.

Internal and external obliques
These two muscle groups wrap your torso from your ribs and spine to your hips, enabling you to bend and twist while supporting your pelvis and spine.

Illiopsoas (Hip Flexor)
These muscles make it possible to flex your thigh at the hip—a key movement for athletic performance.

Adductors
This group of muscles (the adductor brevis, longus, and magnus; pectineus; and gracilis) is collectively responsible for allowing you to pull your leg back toward your body's midline.

Abductors
These include the gluteus medius and minimus as well as the tensor fascia latae and the sartorius. They enable you to move your thigh away from your body.

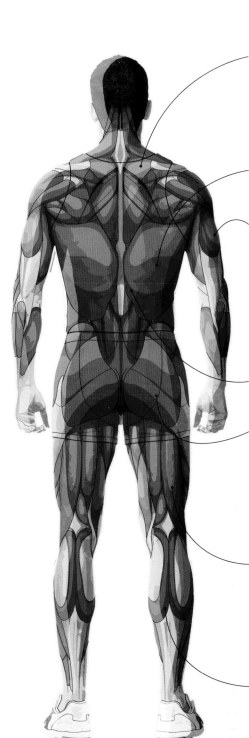

Trapezius
Located at the top of your back and neck, this muscle moves your shoulder blades, particularly during shrugging motions.

Latissimus dorsi
This largest muscle of the back plays a significant role during pulling movements, particularly when pulling your arms toward your body's midline, like when doing a pullup.

Triceps
This three-headed muscle runs along the back of your upper arm between your shoulder and elbow. It's responsible for bending your elbow.

Erector spinae
These muscles run the entire length of your spine and are credited with keeping your back straight as well as assisting with spinal rotation.

Gluteals
Together, the gluteus maximus, gluteus minimus, and gluteus medius make up the strong, powerful muscles of your butt. They work to move your hips and thighs— most often in conjunction with other muscle groups.

Hamstrings
Working as the counterbalance to your quads, the three muscles of the hamstrings—the semitendinosus, the semimembranosus, and the biceps femoris—work together to flex your knees and lift your hips.

Calves
The two major muscles of your lower legs—the gastrocnemius and the soleus—are what make it possible to plant your foot and push off the ground.

WHAT'S YOUR "CORE"?

The term *core* gets thrown around a lot in fitness, and it's often thought of as a synonym for "abs," but that's not really the case. The core actually consists of all the muscles between your hips and your shoulders, particularly those responsible for stabilizing and supporting the pelvis and thorax (your chest cavity).

When you *engage your core*— another common phrase— you're strengthening the stabilizing muscles of your hips, abs, back, and shoulders while also using your chest, back, and neck to support the exercise. Why is *core* such a fitness buzzword? A strong core is associated with good posture and a lower risk of injury during exercise. It's also a key factor for preventing and reducing lower-back pain.

FUN FACT

Just because certain exercises target specific muscle groups doesn't mean you aren't putting more of your muscles to work. In fact, to take a single step, you use 200 different muscles.

BASIC POSITIONS

Almost all exercises start with a basic starting position or incorporate a basic movement. By mastering these positions and movements, you can quickly, effectively, and safely do almost any exercise in this book. Knowing the correct form for each position is essential to enjoying an effective and safe routine.

SQUAT

A squat is one of the easiest exercises to perform incorrectly. Even if you think you know how to do a squat, double check your form before proceeding. Remember: Initiate the move by pushing your hips backward, not by bending your knees. This helps keep your weight centered over your heels.

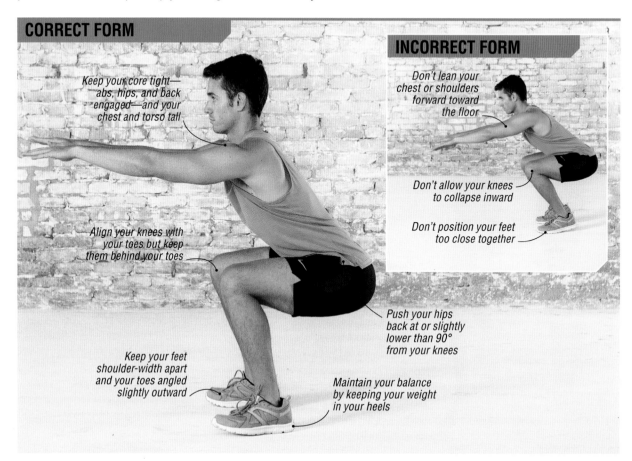

CORRECT FORM

Keep your core tight—abs, hips, and back engaged—and your chest and torso tall

Align your knees with your toes but keep them behind your toes

Keep your feet shoulder-width apart and your toes angled slightly outward

Maintain your balance by keeping your weight in your heels

INCORRECT FORM

Don't lean your chest or shoulders forward toward the floor

Don't allow your knees to collapse inward

Don't position your feet too close together

Push your hips back at or slightly lower than 90° from your knees

LUNGE

The lunge, like the squat, is often performed incorrectly. By mastering the correct lunge form, you can feel confident performing more challenging lunge exercises with a reduced risk of injury.

CORRECT FORM

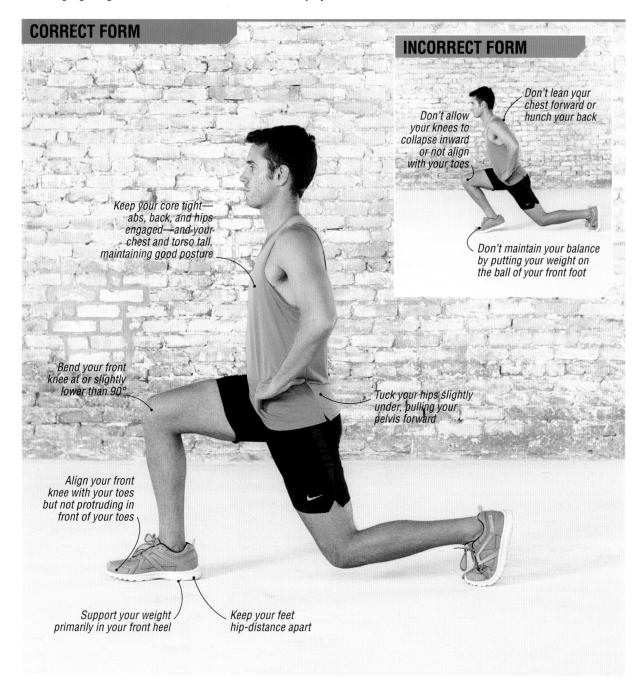

INCORRECT FORM

Don't lean your chest forward or hunch your back

Don't allow your knees to collapse inward or not align with your toes

Don't maintain your balance by putting your weight on the ball of your front foot

Keep your core tight—abs, back, and hips engaged—and your chest and torso tall, maintaining good posture

Bend your front knee at or slightly lower than 90°

Tuck your hips slightly under, pulling your pelvis forward

Align your front knee with your toes but not protruding in front of your toes

Support your weight primarily in your front heel

Keep your feet hip-distance apart

DEFENSIVE STANCE

The defensive stance—or the athletic stance—is a basic position that prepares you to move quickly in any direction. It's often the starting position for active exercises, and it's a stance used in many different sports.

CORRECT FORM

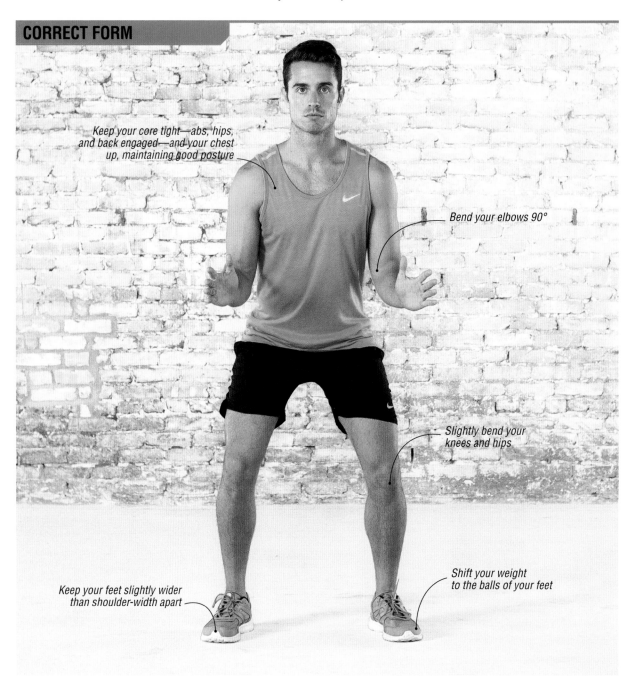

Keep your core tight—abs, hips, and back engaged—and your chest up, maintaining good posture

Bend your elbows 90°

Slightly bend your knees and hips

Keep your feet slightly wider than shoulder-width apart

Shift your weight to the balls of your feet

HIGH PLANK

Correct form for the high plank is identical to correct form for starting a pushup—
your arms straight, core tight, holding your torso away from the floor. If you can do
the high plank correctly, then you can also master a pushup.

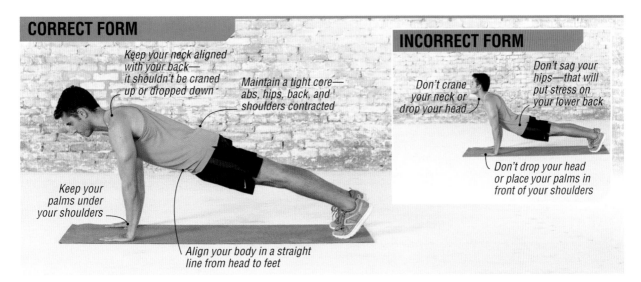

CORRECT FORM

Keep your neck aligned
with your back—
it shouldn't be craned
up or dropped down

Maintain a tight core—
abs, hips, back, and
shoulders contracted

Keep your
palms under
your shoulders

Align your body in a straight
line from head to feet

INCORRECT FORM

Don't crane
your neck or
drop your head

Don't sag your
hips—that will
put stress on
your lower back

Don't drop your head
or place your palms in
front of your shoulders

BOTTOM OF A PUSHUP

The bottom of the pushup is when mistakes often happen, particularly
when you lower yourself to the floor and push yourself back up again.
Pay attention to the alignment of your spine and neck during this transition.

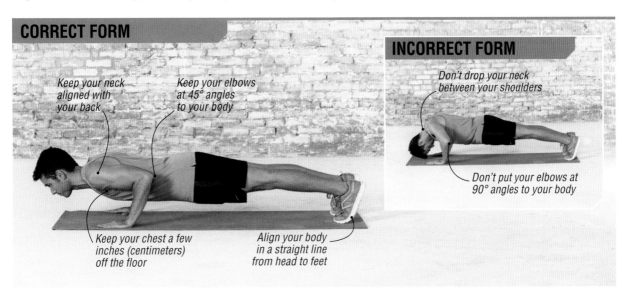

CORRECT FORM

Keep your neck
aligned with
your back

Keep your elbows
at 45° angles
to your body

Keep your chest a few
inches (centimeters)
off the floor

Align your body
in a straight line
from head to feet

INCORRECT FORM

Don't drop your neck
between your shoulders

Don't put your elbows at
90° angles to your body

WARMING UP

Starting a tough routine without warming up is like taking a test without studying—almost nothing good can come from it. A warmup enables your core temperature to gradually rise as your heart starts pumping more blood and oxygen to working muscles. Ultimately, this prepares you for exercise and helps prevent injuries. Do all five warmups in order.

POTATO SACK LUNGES

You'll move in sync with your partner as you perform this exercise—almost as if you were in a three-legged race. Make sure to constantly communicate with your partner to stay on track.

1 Stand shoulder to shoulder with your partner, wrapping your inside arm around her shoulder or hip. Moving your inside legs in tandem, step forward together to perform a lunge.

2 Push through your front heels to rise to standing, lifting your outside legs as you step forward and planting your heels to lunge again. Keep alternating steps for 1 minute.

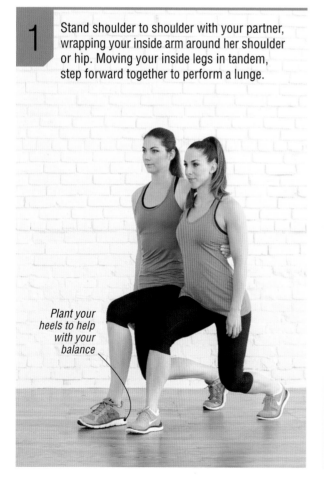

Plant your heels to help with your balance

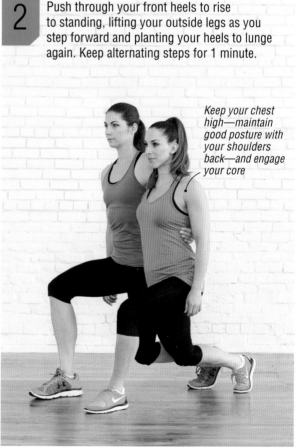

Keep your chest high—maintain good posture with your shoulders back—and engage your core

PLANK QUICK FEET

This warmup exercise will engage one partner in a static plank while the other partner actively jogs back and forth across her partner's legs. This action increases your heart rate and helps prepare you for more strenuous work.

1 Stand between your partner's feet in a defensive stance. Hop over your partner's right calf, landing on your right foot.

Start in the high plank position, with your shoulders over your palms and your body straight. Position your feet about hip-distance apart.

Once you land, draw your left foot into the air as if jogging in place

Keep your weight in the balls of your feet throughout

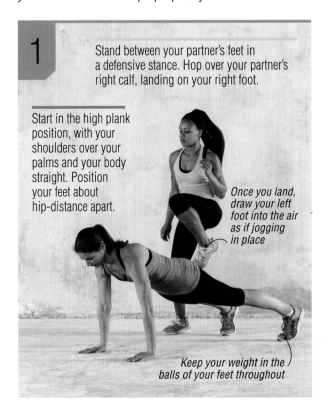

2 Immediately set your left foot back down between your partner's legs, and hop your right foot back to center.

Maintain your high plank position.

If your high plank becomes too challenging, you can lower your knees to the floor

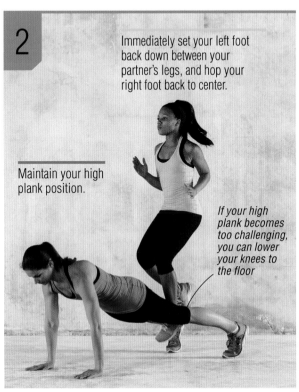

3 Each partner should perform both parts of the exercise twice, rotating back and forth every 60 seconds.

Continue to maintain your high plank position.

Stay light on your feet, and pump your arms

Perform the quick feet to the opposite side, hopping your left foot over your partner's left calf and planting the ball of your foot before you lift your right foot into the air, as if jogging.

Perform all the hops as quickly as possible, but if the best you can do is step over your partner, that's fine

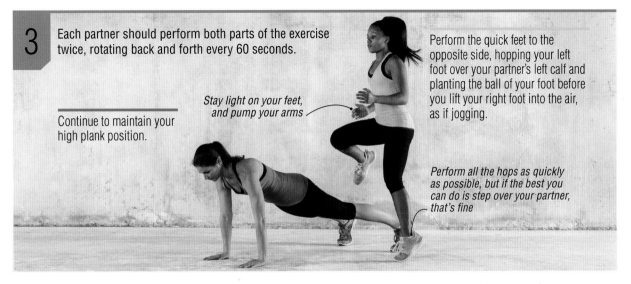

DOWNWARD DOG & BEAR CRAWL

During this exercise, you'll combine an active stretch with a demanding cardio-focused exercise that challenges your shoulders, chest, quads, and glutes. You'll constantly change roles, ensuring each partner has a chance to warm up the same muscle groups.

1

Keep your neck aligned with your back, and don't allow your head to crane

Start on your hands and knees—perpendicular to your partner—with your feet flexed and your toes tucked under so the balls of your feet are on the floor.

Lift your knees off the floor, using your hands and the balls of your feet to help you find your initial balance

Start in the high plank position.

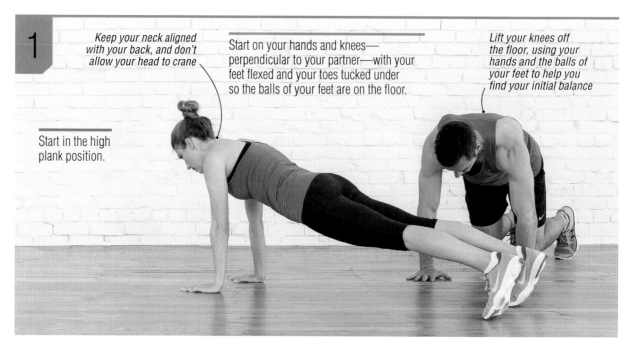

2

Keeping your knees off the floor, crawl forward—the *bear crawl*—and under your partner's downward dog.

Push your hips upward, pushing through your palms and feet until your body forms an inverted V. This is a stance called a *downward dog*.

Push your heels down for a deeper stretch, but they don't need to touch the floor

If you're having a hard time fitting under your partner, lower your belly to the floor and use your arms to pull yourself under your partner

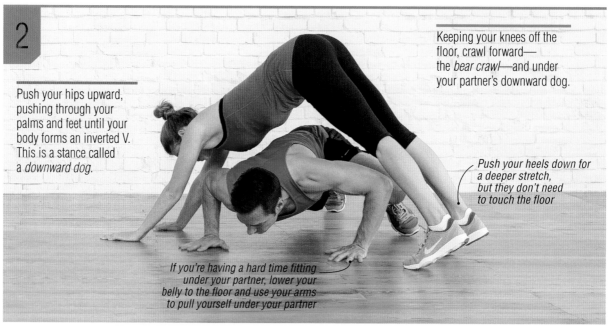

3

After crawling under your partner, rotate 90° and straighten into the high plank position.

After your partner crawls under you, lower back to your original high plank and rotate 90° toward your partner, setting up in the bear crawl position.

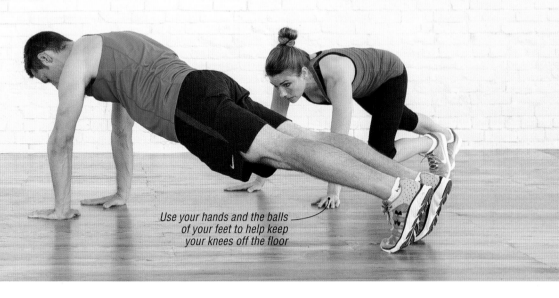

Use your hands and the balls of your feet to help keep your knees off the floor

4

After setting up in the high plank, push through your palms and the balls of your feet as you lift your hips toward the sky and into an inverted V position. Perform this exercise for 1 minute, continuing to switch roles.

When your partner gets into a downward dog, crawl forward under your partner's body, keeping your knees off the floor.

VARIATION

If space is limited, reverse this exercise after performing a repetition, and crawl backward under your partner before switching roles.

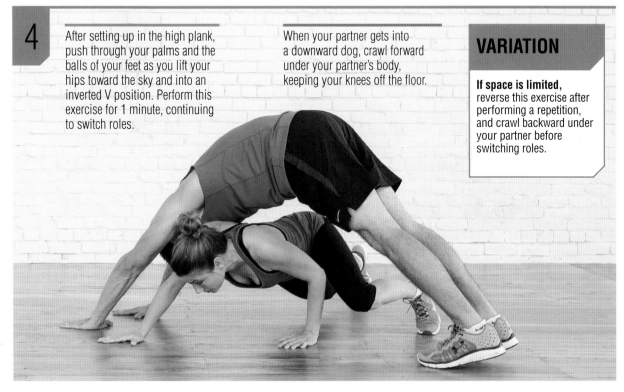

LEAP FROGS

As you perform the warmup exercises provided in this book, always do this one last—just before you start your regular workout routine. It's the most strenuous of the bunch, and the other warmup exercises will prepare you to perform the plyometric jump.

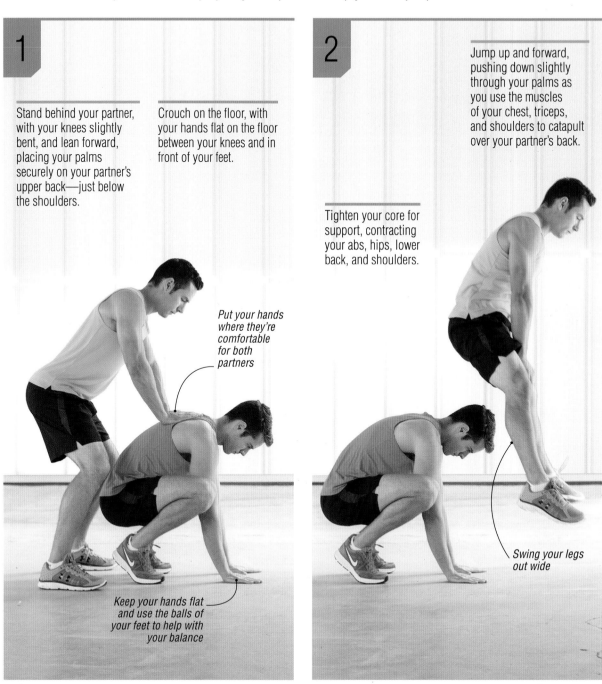

1

Stand behind your partner, with your knees slightly bent, and lean forward, placing your palms securely on your partner's upper back—just below the shoulders.

Crouch on the floor, with your hands flat on the floor between your knees and in front of your feet.

Put your hands where they're comfortable for both partners

Keep your hands flat and use the balls of your feet to help with your balance

2

Jump up and forward, pushing down slightly through your palms as you use the muscles of your chest, triceps, and shoulders to catapult over your partner's back.

Tighten your core for support, contracting your abs, hips, lower back, and shoulders.

Swing your legs out wide

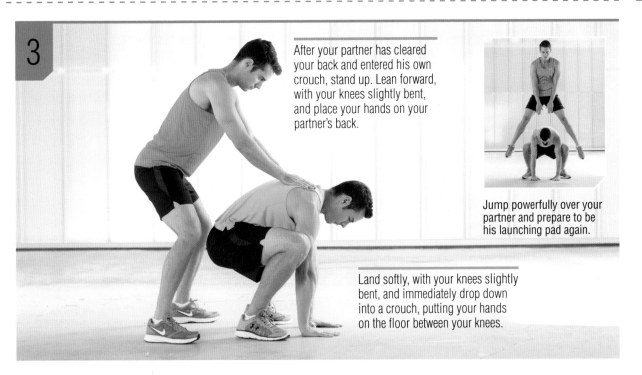

3 After your partner has cleared your back and entered his own crouch, stand up. Lean forward, with your knees slightly bent, and place your hands on your partner's back.

Jump powerfully over your partner and prepare to be his launching pad again.

Land softly, with your knees slightly bent, and immediately drop down into a crouch, putting your hands on the floor between your knees.

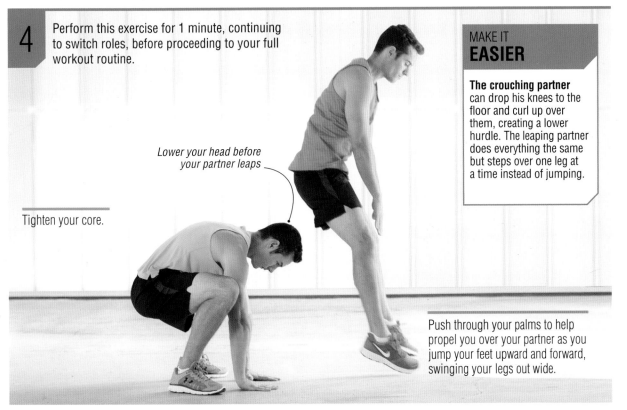

4 Perform this exercise for 1 minute, continuing to switch roles, before proceeding to your full workout routine.

Lower your head before your partner leaps

Tighten your core.

MAKE IT EASIER

The crouching partner can drop his knees to the floor and curl up over them, creating a lower hurdle. The leaping partner does everything the same but steps over one leg at a time instead of jumping.

Push through your palms to help propel you over your partner as you jump your feet upward and forward, swinging your legs out wide.

COOLING DOWN

Flexibility is one of the five components of fitness, making it an extremely important (albeit often overlooked) part of a workout program. When you use stretching as part of your post-workout cooldown, your muscles are already warm and pliable, making it easier to maintain—or even increase—your range of motion through your major joints.

FORWARD FOLD

You'll stretch the entire back of your body—your calves, hamstrings, glutes, and back—with this exercise. If keeping your legs straight is too challenging, perform this exercise with a slight bend in your knees.

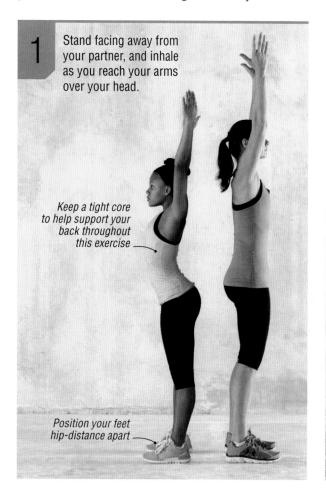

1 Stand facing away from your partner, and inhale as you reach your arms over your head.

Keep a tight core to help support your back throughout this exercise

Position your feet hip-distance apart

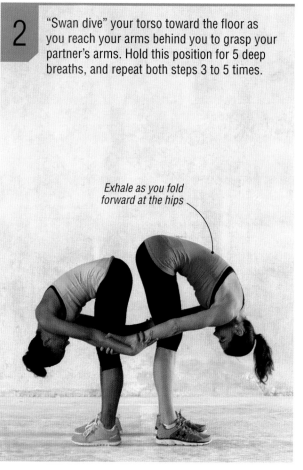

2 "Swan dive" your torso toward the floor as you reach your arms behind you to grasp your partner's arms. Hold this position for 5 deep breaths, and repeat both steps 3 to 5 times.

Exhale as you fold forward at the hips

CHILD'S POSE & BACKBEND

This stretch should feel relaxing for both partners—with one partner enjoying a lengthening stretch of the spine and shoulders while the other partner enjoys a heart-opening backbend that stretches out the shoulders and chest as well as the hip flexors and core.

1

Kneel on the floor, sitting on your heels. Fold over your legs, reaching your arms forward as you relax into the stretch. This is the child's pose. Take 2 deep breaths.

When your partner is in the child's pose, sit lightly on her tailbone—tailbone to tailbone—using your hands to help push her hips down farther.

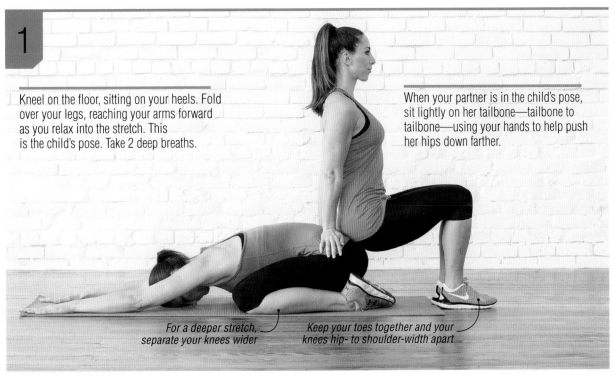

For a deeper stretch, separate your knees wider

Keep your toes together and your knees hip- to shoulder-width apart

2 Perform each half of the stretch twice, alternating positions.

Remain in the child's pose, breathing deeply. Communicate with your partner regarding your comfort level.

Lean back, aligning your spine with your partner's until you're completely straight. Reach your arms back and behind your head. Take 5 deep breaths.

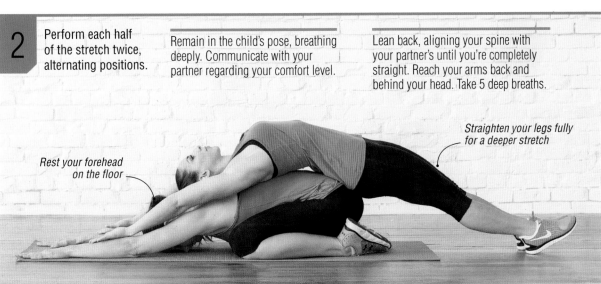

Straighten your legs fully for a deeper stretch

Rest your forehead on the floor

STRADDLE & PULL

This is another great stretch for your hamstrings, adductors, and lower back as it helps increase your flexibility by targeting the adductor muscles of your inner thighs while also offering a lengthening stretch of the spine and hamstrings. Move slowly to prevent overstretching.

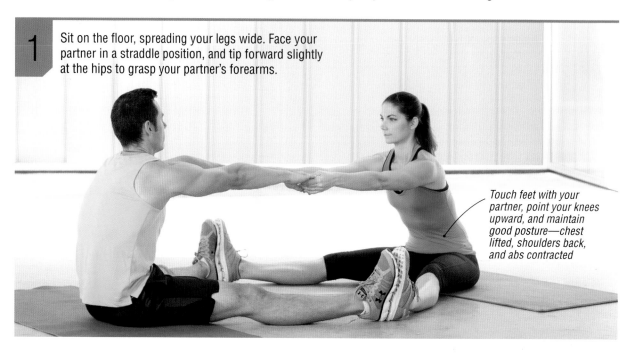

1 Sit on the floor, spreading your legs wide. Face your partner in a straddle position, and tip forward slightly at the hips to grasp your partner's forearms.

Touch feet with your partner, point your knees upward, and maintain good posture—chest lifted, shoulders back, and abs contracted

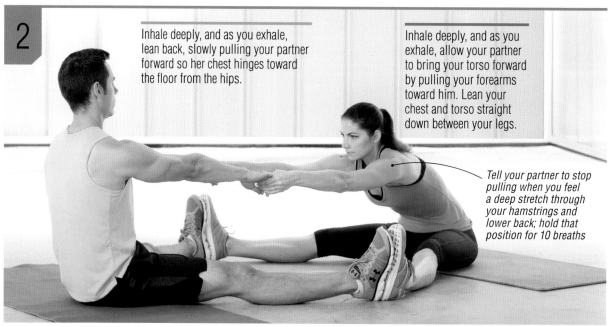

2 Inhale deeply, and as you exhale, lean back, slowly pulling your partner forward so her chest hinges toward the floor from the hips.

Inhale deeply, and as you exhale, allow your partner to bring your torso forward by pulling your forearms toward him. Lean your chest and torso straight down between your legs.

Tell your partner to stop pulling when you feel a deep stretch through your hamstrings and lower back; hold that position for 10 breaths

STANDING FIGURE 4 HIP STRETCH

For a deep stretch of your glutes and hips, try this exercise.
The movement does require balance and coordination,
but it's easier to perform with a partner than on your own.

1 Stand facing your partner. Reach forward, grasping your partner's wrists or forearms. Lift your left foot off the floor and place your left ankle across your right thigh in a 4 shape.

2 Push your hips backward, bending your supporting knee and lowering yourself into a modified squat. You should feel a stretch through the outside of your left hip and glute.

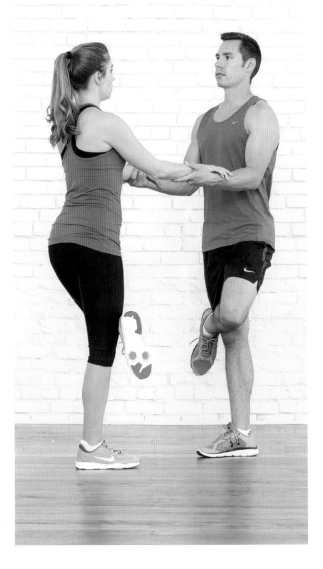

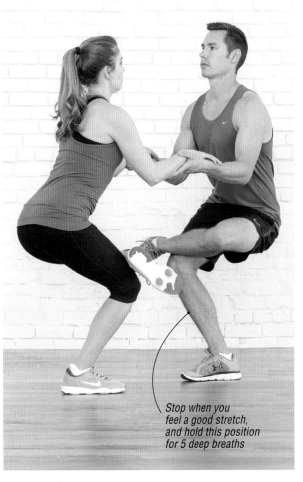

Stop when you feel a good stretch, and hold this position for 5 deep breaths

RECOVERY

Stretching isn't the only way to maximize your post-workout routine. To enhance recovery, it's important to consider hydration, nutrition, and self-massage.

HYDRATION

All your cellular functions take place in the medium of water. If your cells are dehydrated, your body can't effectively work on all cylinders. The result is a slowed metabolism and hindered repair of muscle tissue because your body isn't able to deliver key nutrients or remove waste products from your cells as quickly as it could if it were fully hydrated.

When you hydrate appropriately after your workout by topping off your water stores, your cells are able to recover and repair at an optimum speed. This actually helps prepare you for your next workout so you can hit the gym feeling your absolute best.

No Need for Sports Drinks

Replace the *extras* in sports drinks—glucose (sugar) and electrolytes (mostly sodium and potassium)—with post-workout meals. You don't lose enough of them to need to replace them with fluids.

WATER INTAKE

These general guidelines apply to most workouts, but when exercising in hot and humid environments or at high levels of intensity, increase your fluid intake.

BEFORE WORKOUTS

Drink about 16 ounces (500ml) of water 2 hours before beginning an exercise.

DURING WORKOUTS

Every 15–20 minutes, take a break to drink 4–6 ounces (120 to 180ml) of water.

AFTER WORKOUTS

Slowly drink about 1 to 2 quarts (1 to 2L) of water over the next few hours to replace fluid loss.

FOAM ROLLING

Massages loosen up knots while supporting the delivery of key nutrients to muscle fibers and clearing away waste. If you don't have a massage therapist at your beck and call, a foam roller is the next best thing.

1 Roll a muscle group slowly over the hard foam cylinder.

2 When you find a tight spot, stop rolling and move lightly across the knot to help loosen the adhesion.

3 Repeat steps 1 and 2 to perform roughly 10 passes across a muscle group.

GLUTE ROLLOUT

Sit on the roller, with your hands on the floor behind you. Cross your legs, putting weight on your lifted glute. Roll across the roller. Switch sides after 10 passes.

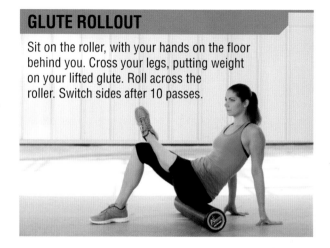

NUTRITION

Tough workouts are catabolic: They break down larger molecules to create energy for movement. If you don't refuel properly, the energy requirements for recovery continue this activity, which can lead to undesirable outcomes: glycogen depletion and muscle wasting.

If you ate about an hour before exercise, the nutrients will help carry you post-workout. Aim to eat within 2 hours after your workout—either a regularly scheduled meal or a small meal or snack to aid in recovery before your next full meal.

BALANCED PROTEIN–CARBOHYDRATE MEALS

A protein- and carbohydrate-rich meal in a ratio roughly 4:1, like one of those listed, eaten shortly after exercise will provide your body with the nutrients it needs to recover and repair.

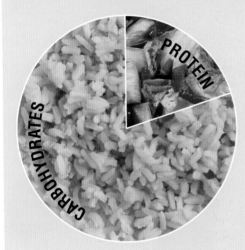

- **Yogurt parfait:** 8 ounces (225g) of Greek yogurt with 8 ounces (225g) of blueberries, 1 tablespoon of honey, and 2 ounces (5g) of walnuts
- **Chocolate milk (use whole milk):** 8 ounces (225ml)
- **Tuna salad sandwich and a medium banana:** 2 ounces of tuna, 1 TB. of mayonnaise, 1 TB. of sweet pickle relish, and 2 slices of whole wheat bread
- **Chicken stir fry over rice:** 6 ounces (170g) of chicken/veggie stir fry and 1 cup of brown rice

- **Egg sandwich:** 2 cooked eggs, 6 leaves of fresh spinach, and 1 slice of tomato on 2 slices of whole wheat bread
- **Spaghetti:** 4 ounces (113g) of spaghetti with $1/3$ cup of tomato-based meat sauce
- **Turkey wrap and $1/2$ cup of baby carrots:** 2 ounces of turkey rolled inside a wheat wrap, with $1/2$ cup of avocado, 2 TB. of hummus, and as many fresh veggies as you like
- **Bagel:** 1 bagel with 2 TB. of peanut butter and 1 TB. of jelly
- **Cereal:** $1 1/2$ cups of dry cereal and 8 ounces (225g) of whole milk
- **Trail mix:** $1/3$ cup of trail mix
- **Protein bar**

MID- TO UPPER-BACK ROLLOUT

Lie on the roller so it's positioned perpendicularly at the middle of your back. Lift your hips and slowly roll up and down atop the roller from your middle to upper back. Do this for 10 passes.

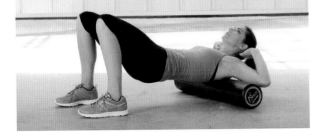

QUAD ROLLOUT

Balance on your forearms, with the roller under your quads. Roll slowly over the roller from above your knees to just below your hips: 10 passes each with your toes pointing straight back, out, and in.

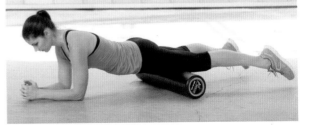

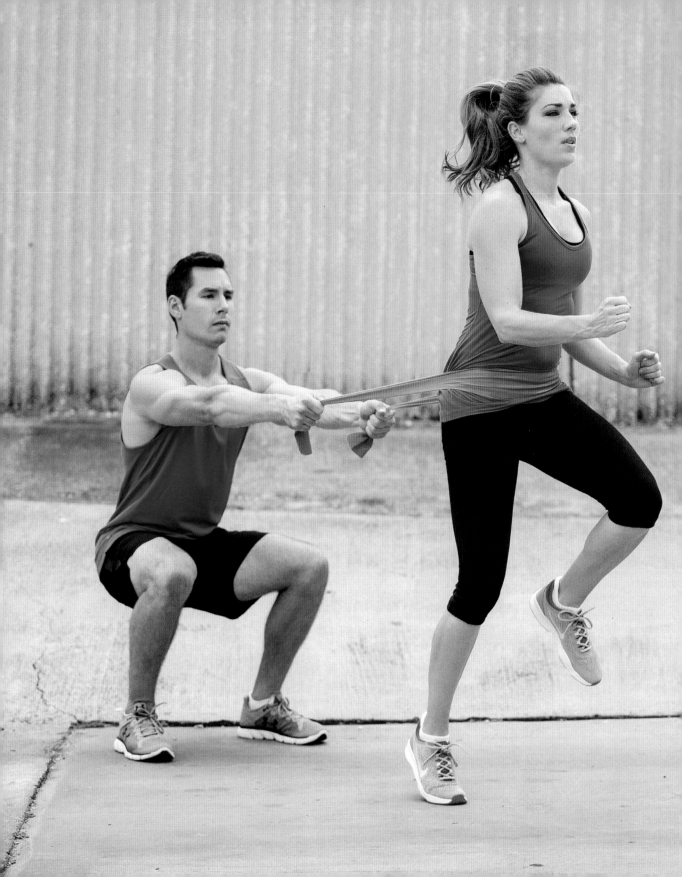

2
RESISTANCE EXERCISES

You'll develop strength, power, speed, and agility while performing these resistance exercises with your partner. Many of these moves use specific equipment to allow you to target different muscle groups, helping you develop greater total-body strength.

LEVEL 1

SQUAT & RESISTANCE BAND SPRINT

REQUIRED EQUIPMENT **RESISTANCE BAND**

This exercise combines lower-body resistance training with cardio, as one partner performs an isometric squat and the other sprints forward. It's important to hold the resistance band tightly, as resisting the sprinter's action makes this exercise more challenging for both partners.

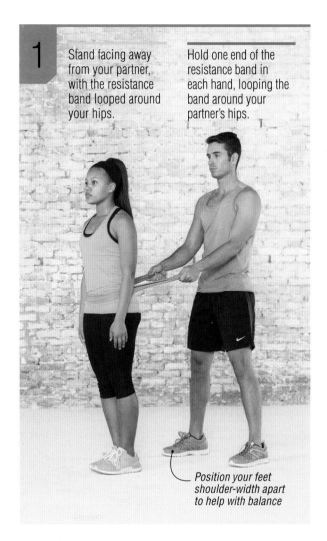

1 Stand facing away from your partner, with the resistance band looped around your hips.

Hold one end of the resistance band in each hand, looping the band around your partner's hips.

Position your feet shoulder-width apart to help with balance

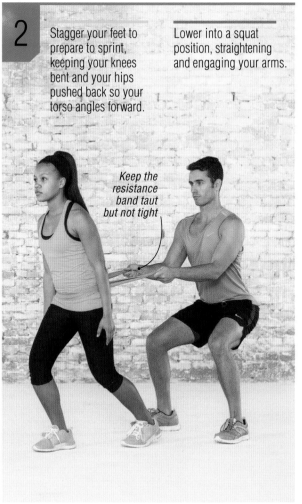

2 Stagger your feet to prepare to sprint, keeping your knees bent and your hips pushed back so your torso angles forward.

Lower into a squat position, straightening and engaging your arms.

Keep the resistance band taut but not tight

3 Keep performing this step for the time listed in the workout or as desired.

Sprint forward quickly until the resistance band prevents you from running farther, and pump your arms and legs to sprint in place.

MAKE IT
HARDER

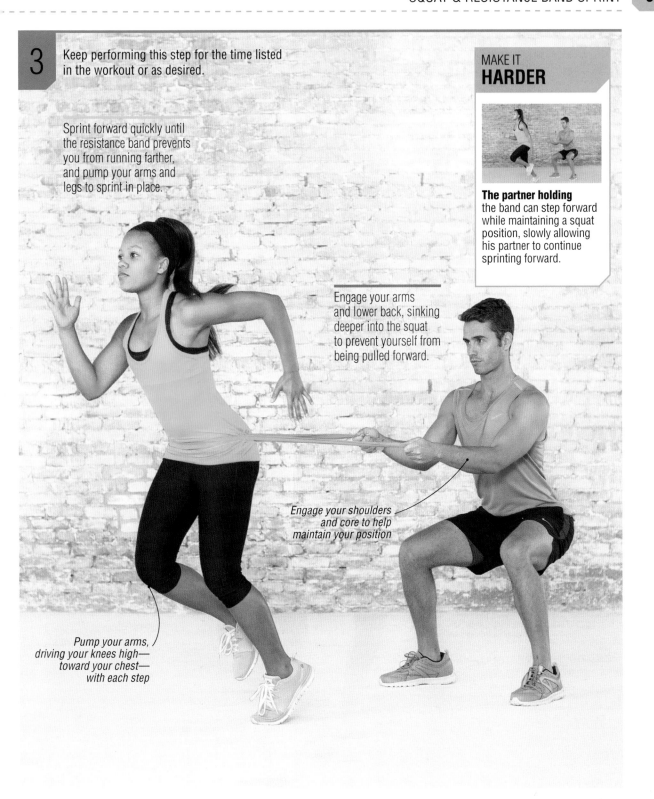

The partner holding the band can step forward while maintaining a squat position, slowly allowing his partner to continue sprinting forward.

Engage your arms and lower back, sinking deeper into the squat to prevent yourself from being pulled forward.

Engage your shoulders and core to help maintain your position

Pump your arms, driving your knees high— toward your chest— with each step

SIDE LUNGE & TWIST

REQUIRED EQUIPMENT **RESISTANCE BAND**

This exercise adds variety to your leg routines with lateral steps that engage your quads, glutes, and inner and outer thighs. The resistance band twist fires up your core, engaging your abs, lower back, hips, and shoulders. The constant movement keeps your heart rate up.

1 Stand side by side with your partner, holding one end of the resistance band at your navel with both hands.

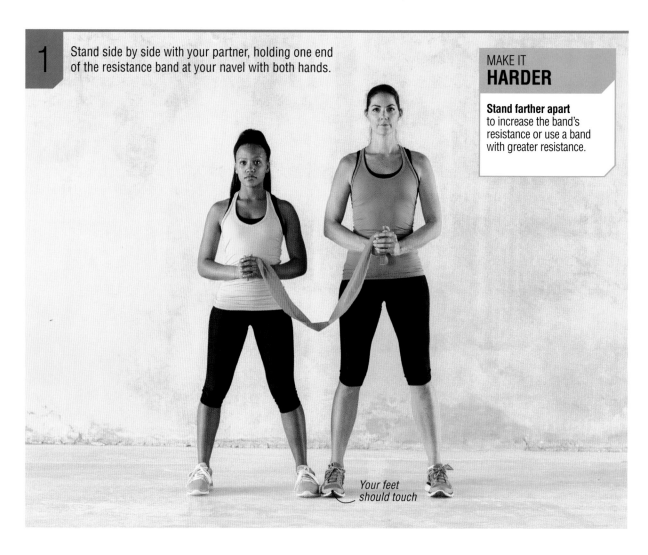

Your feet should touch

MAKE IT HARDER

Stand farther apart to increase the band's resistance or use a band with greater resistance.

2 Using your exterior leg to take a wide step outward, sink into a side lunge by bending your outside knee, keeping it aligned with that foot and pushing your hips back.

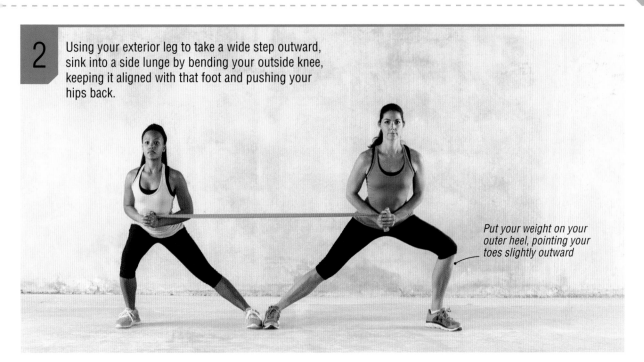

Put your weight on your outer heel, pointing your toes slightly outward

3 Twist your torso to the outside during the lowest point in the lunge, engaging your hips, lower back, abs, and shoulders while keeping your lower body steady.

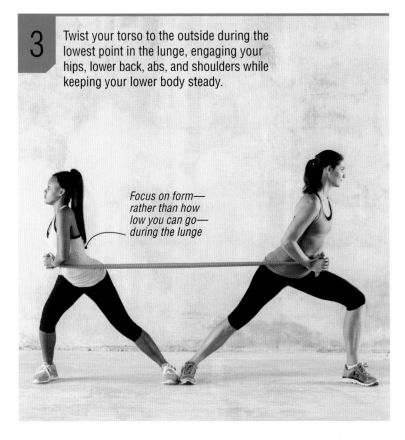

Focus on form—rather than how low you can go—during the lunge

4 Step back to your starting position. Repeat steps 2 to 4 for the time listed in the workout or as desired.

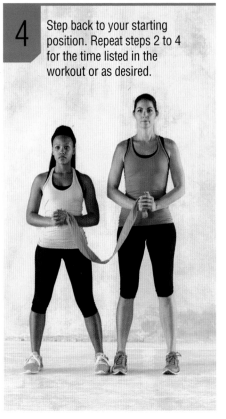

LEVEL 1

SUPERMAN LATS & BICEPS CURLS

REQUIRED EQUIPMENT **RESISTANCE BAND**

Who says you need a gym to work your back? With help from your partner and a resistance band, you can target your lats while simultaneously strengthening your lower back. Plus, you'll have a chance to work your biceps when you switch roles with your partner.

1 Each partner waits until the other has completed her motions before performing her own movements.

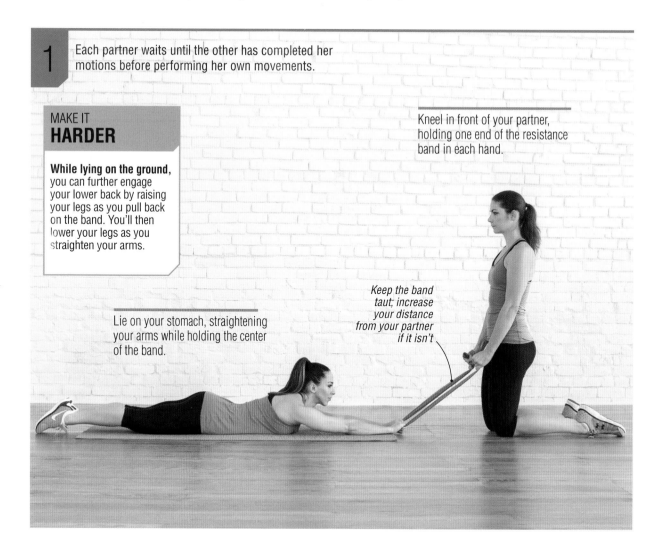

MAKE IT
HARDER

While lying on the ground, you can further engage your lower back by raising your legs as you pull back on the band. You'll then lower your legs as you straighten your arms.

Kneel in front of your partner, holding one end of the resistance band in each hand.

Keep the band taut; increase your distance from your partner if it isn't

Lie on your stomach, straightening your arms while holding the center of the band.

2 Lift your chest off the ground, and bend your elbows to pull the resistance band toward your shoulders.

Pull firmly to provide consistent resistance

Engage your back by pulling your shoulder blades together

Pull back on the band as your partner pulls it toward her chest. Although she controls the movement, you should keep providing resistance.

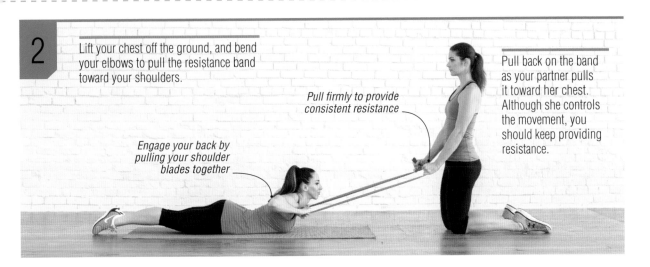

3 Straighten your arms forward, using your core and your lower back to keep your shoulders lifted.

Keep your body steady—don't lean back as you perform the curl

Engaging your core and lower back helps keep your shoulders lifted

Hold your elbows at your sides, engaging your biceps by curling your hands toward your shoulders while pulling against the band's resistance.

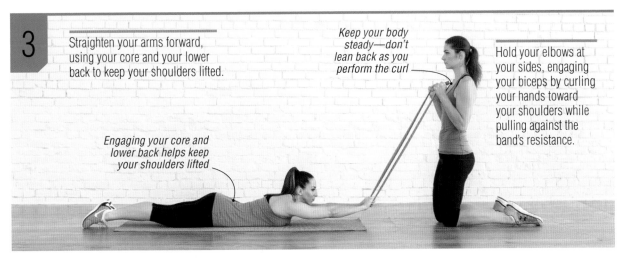

4 Repeat steps 2 to 4 for the time listed in the workout or as desired.

Return to your starting position.

Lower your hands to their starting positions.

Keep your elbows tight against your sides

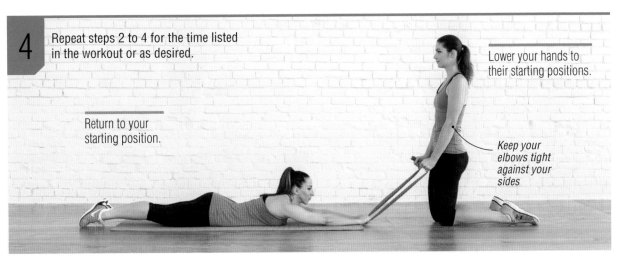

REVERSE LUNGE & TRICEPS EXTENSION

REQUIRED EQUIPMENT **2 RESISTANCE BANDS WITH EQUAL RESISTANCE**

While the reverse lunges will challenge your lower body, the extensions will isolate and strengthen the muscles running along the backs of your upper arms. Just make sure the two resistance bands you use offer equal resistance because you don't want to work one arm more than the other.

1 Stand across from your partner, holding one end of each resistance band in each hand.

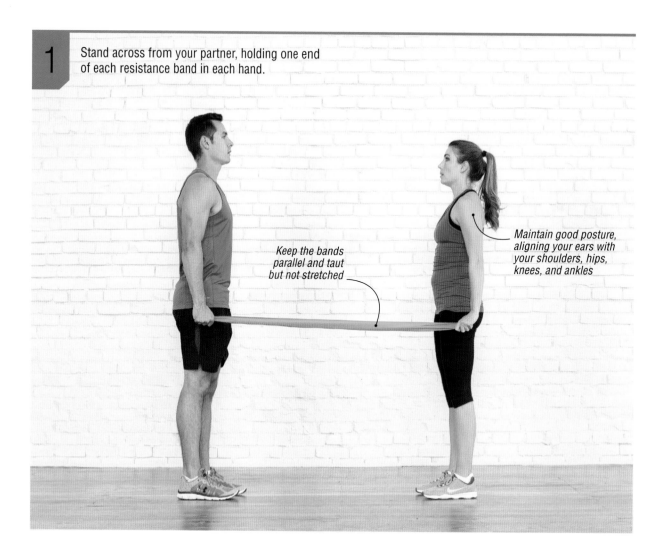

Keep the bands parallel and taut but not stretched

Maintain good posture, aligning your ears with your shoulders, hips, knees, and ankles

2 Step backward with your right leg to perform a reverse lunge. Lower your right knee toward the floor, simultaneously contracting your triceps as you pull your arms straight back against the bands' resistance.

VARIATION

Replace the lunge with a curtsy lunge by crossing your back leg behind your front one so your knees are one behind the other.

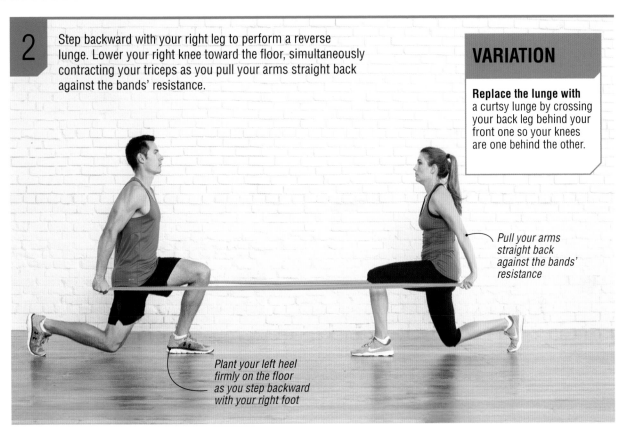

Pull your arms straight back against the bands' resistance

Plant your left heel firmly on the floor as you step backward with your right foot

3 Push through your front heel, and step your back leg forward to stand again.

4 Step back with your left leg to perform a reverse lunge, contracting your triceps and pulling your arms straight back against the bands' resistance.

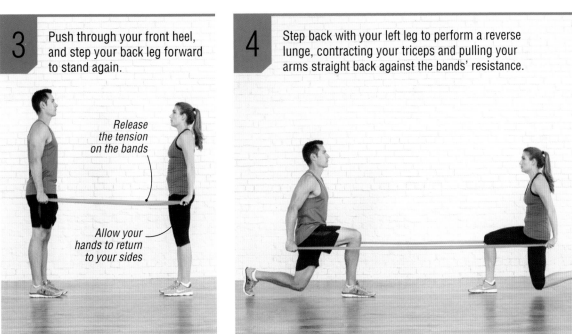

Release the tension on the bands

Allow your hands to return to your sides

WEIGHTED PLANK & DUMBBELL ROW

REQUIRED EQUIPMENT **DUMBBELL**

During this exercise, one partner acts as a bench and the other partner uses that bench for support to complete the dumbbell row, targeting the upper back. When you're the one in the plank position, you have the added challenge of supporting your partner's weight.

1

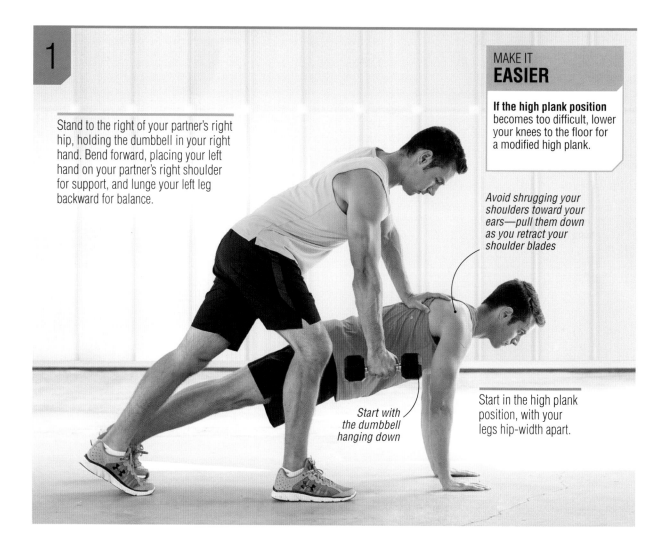

Stand to the right of your partner's right hip, holding the dumbbell in your right hand. Bend forward, placing your left hand on your partner's right shoulder for support, and lunge your left leg backward for balance.

MAKE IT EASIER

If the high plank position becomes too difficult, lower your knees to the floor for a modified high plank.

Avoid shrugging your shoulders toward your ears—pull them down as you retract your shoulder blades

Start with the dumbbell hanging down

Start in the high plank position, with your legs hip-width apart.

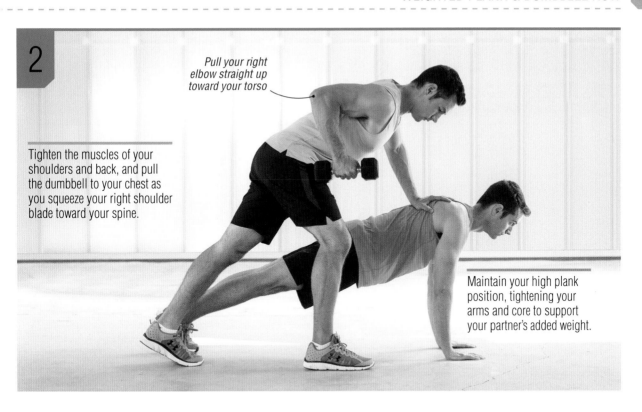

2

Pull your right elbow straight up toward your torso

Tighten the muscles of your shoulders and back, and pull the dumbbell to your chest as you squeeze your right shoulder blade toward your spine.

Maintain your high plank position, tightening your arms and core to support your partner's added weight.

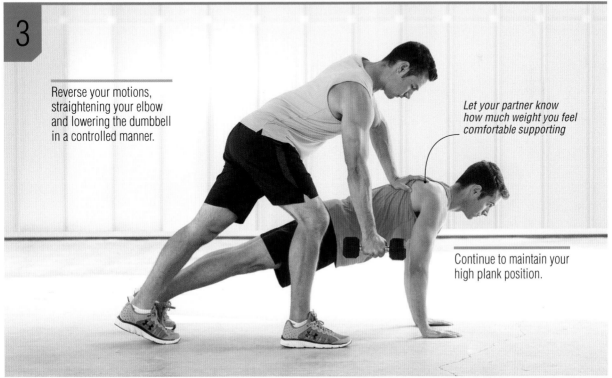

3

Reverse your motions, straightening your elbow and lowering the dumbbell in a controlled manner.

Let your partner know how much weight you feel comfortable supporting

Continue to maintain your high plank position.

WEIGHTED PLANK & TRICEPS EXTENSION

REQUIRED EQUIPMENT **DUMBBELL**

While in one role for this exercise, you'll act as a bench, focusing on the muscles of your core. In the other role, you'll isolate your triceps, strengthening the back of your upper arms as you act as added weight to make your partner's high plank more challenging.

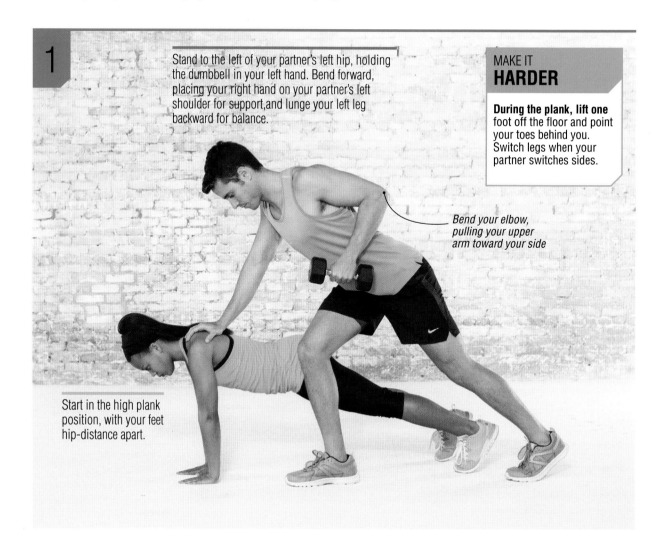

1 Stand to the left of your partner's left hip, holding the dumbbell in your left hand. Bend forward, placing your right hand on your partner's left shoulder for support, and lunge your left leg backward for balance.

MAKE IT
HARDER

During the plank, lift one foot off the floor and point your toes behind you. Switch legs when your partner switches sides.

Bend your elbow, pulling your upper arm toward your side

Start in the high plank position, with your feet hip-distance apart.

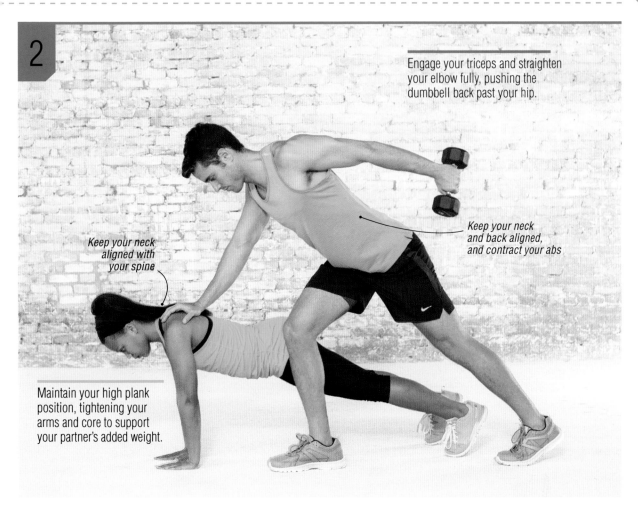

2

Engage your triceps and straighten your elbow fully, pushing the dumbbell back past your hip.

Keep your neck and back aligned, and contract your abs

Keep your neck aligned with your spine

Maintain your high plank position, tightening your arms and core to support your partner's added weight.

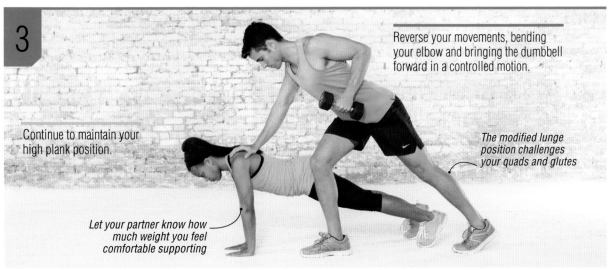

3

Reverse your movements, bending your elbow and bringing the dumbbell forward in a controlled motion.

Continue to maintain your high plank position.

The modified lunge position challenges your quads and glutes

Let your partner know how much weight you feel comfortable supporting

LEVEL 1

RESISTANCE BAND CHEST PRESS & ROW

REQUIRED EQUIPMENT **2 RESISTANCE BANDS WITH EQUAL RESISTANCE**

This exercise targets different muscles groups depending on which role you perform. In one role, you'll work your chest. In the other role, you'll work your upper back. Because both partners are working opposing muscle groups, it's easy to switch roles without rest.

1

Stand facing away from your partner in a defensive stance, holding one end of each resistance band in each hand.

Stand in a defensive stance, facing your partner's back. Hold one end of each resistance band in each hand.

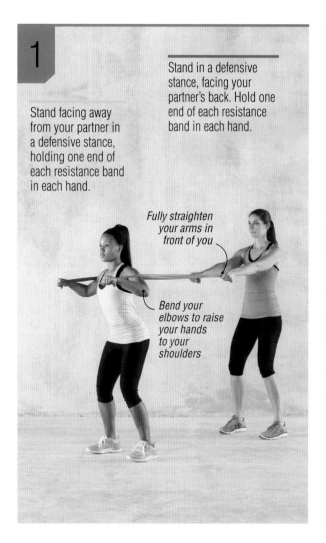

Fully straighten your arms in front of you

Bend your elbows to raise your hands to your shoulders

2

Push your arms straight forward, straightening your elbows at chest height as you push against the resistance.

Pull your arms straight back, bending your elbows and pulling them to your sides against the bands' resistance.

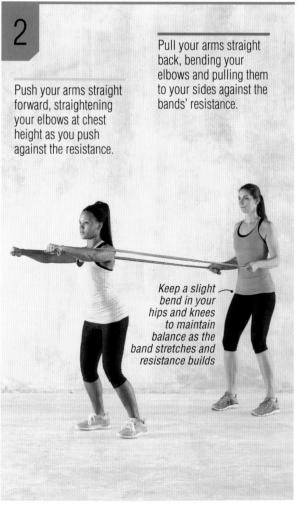

Keep a slight bend in your hips and knees to maintain balance as the band stretches and resistance builds

3

MAKE IT
HARDER

Use resistance bands with a higher level of resistance or start this exercise by standing farther away from your partner.

Control your movements, making sure not to bend your elbows too quickly.

Reverse your movements, straightening your arms in a controlled fashion.

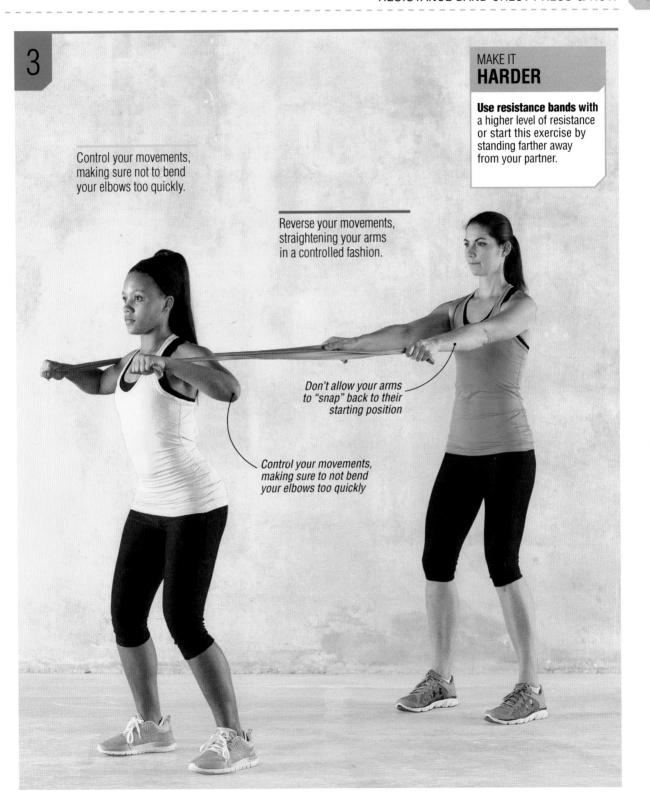

Don't allow your arms to "snap" back to their starting position

Control your movements, making sure to not bend your elbows too quickly

LEVEL 1

SQUAT, REACH & PASS

REQUIRED EQUIPMENT   **MEDICINE BALL**

This full-body exercise is a great way to warm up your legs, glutes, core, and shoulders—all in an effort to get your heart pumping. Just be sure to watch your form—it's tempting to cheat on squats.

1 Start in a defensive stance, facing away from your partner.

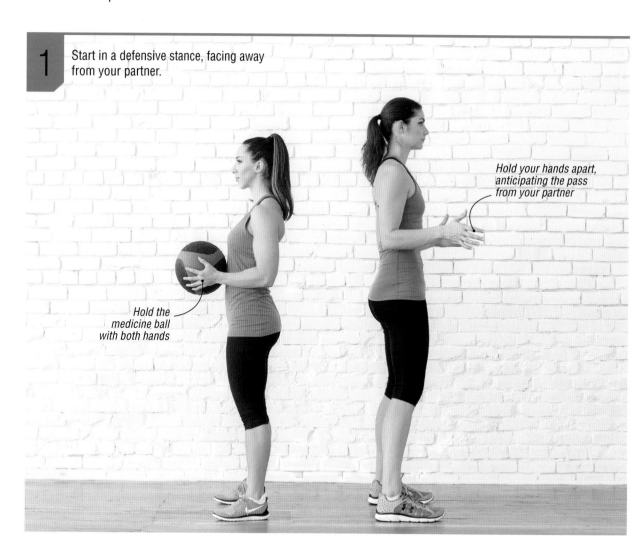

Hold your hands apart, anticipating the pass from your partner

Hold the medicine ball with both hands

2 Squat down, looking up slightly to prevent you from leaning your chest forward toward the floor.

Reach your arms down between your legs to take the ball from your partner.

Pass the ball between your legs to your partner.

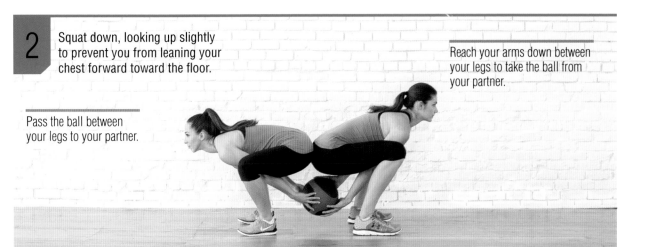

3 Repeat steps 2 and 3 for the time listed in the workouts or as desired.

Don't cheat— reach your arms as high as they'll go

Stand up, reaching your arms over your head and slightly behind you to grab the ball from your partner.

Stand up, lifting the ball over your head and slightly behind you to pass it to your partner.

MAKE IT
HARDER

Use a heavier ball to increase the resistance, making this a total-body challenge. Choose a weight you can lift over your head without fear of dropping it.

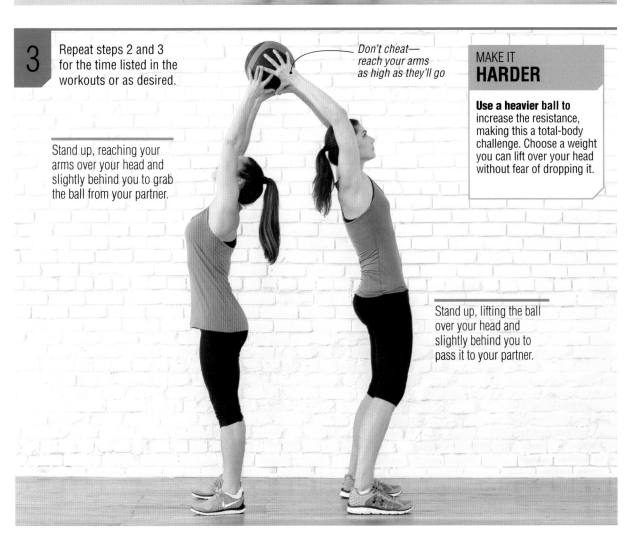

STABILITY BALL SITUP & PASS

REQUIRED EQUIPMENT **STABILITY BALL**

While the stability ball won't add significant weight to this exercise, it does require greater control, encouraging beginners to focus on their abs rather than allowing their momentum to carry them through the movements. For experienced individuals, this exercise offers an effective core warmup.

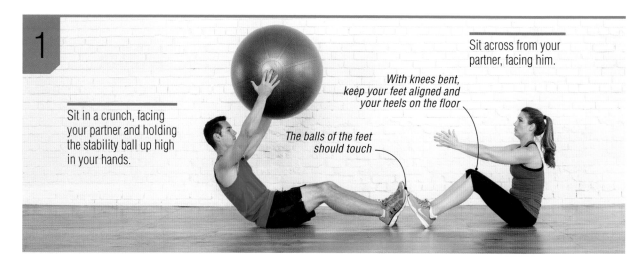

1

Sit in a crunch, facing your partner and holding the stability ball up high in your hands.

With knees bent, keep your feet aligned and your heels on the floor

The balls of the feet should touch

Sit across from your partner, facing him.

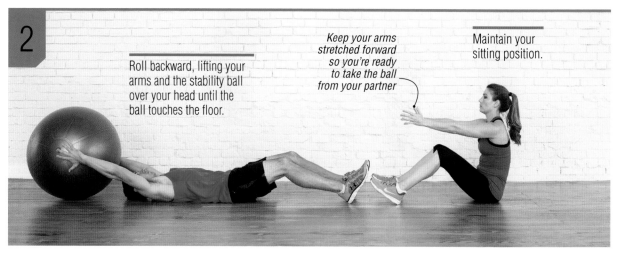

2

Roll backward, lifting your arms and the stability ball over your head until the ball touches the floor.

Keep your arms stretched forward so you're ready to take the ball from your partner

Maintain your sitting position.

3

Take the ball from your partner.

Reverse your motion, using your abs to roll up to a seated position before handing the ball to your partner.

VARIATION

Instead of doing a situp, roll down to a 45° angle, then twist to touch the stability ball to the floor on either side of you before sitting up.

Always keep your glutes firmly on the floor

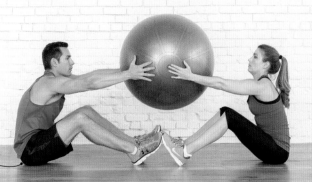

4

Roll backward, lifting your arms and the stability ball over your head until the ball touches the floor.

Maintain your sitting position.

Keep your lower back in contact with the floor as you perform the situp

5

Reverse your motion, using your abs to roll up to a seated position, and hand the stability ball to your partner.

Keep your arms stretched forward to prepare to receive the ball from your partner.

Avoid using momentum to throw yourself forward to a seated position

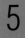
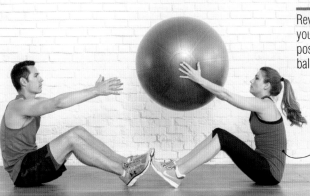

LEVEL 1

SLIDING CHEST PASS

REQUIRED EQUIPMENT **MEDICINE BALL**

Passing a medicine ball back and forth with your partner while performing a lateral (sideways) slide is a great way to increase your heart rate while also strengthening your upper body. Start with a lightweight ball before graduating to a heavier weight.

1 Stand facing your partner in a defensive stance, keeping your knees and elbows bent and your feet shoulder-width apart.

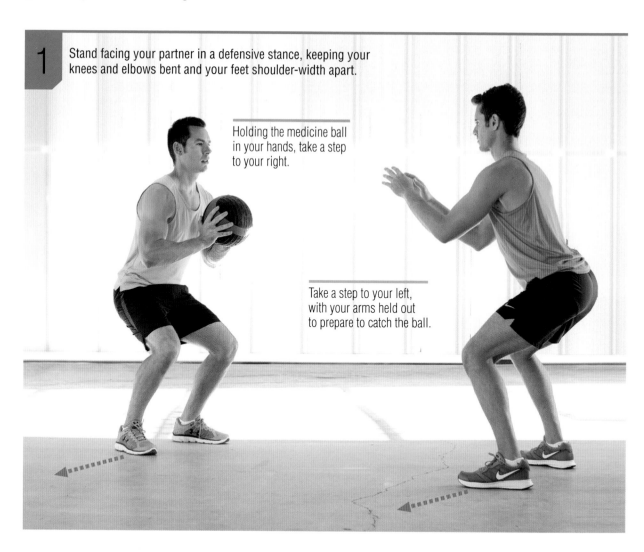

Holding the medicine ball in your hands, take a step to your right.

Take a step to your left, with your arms held out to prepare to catch the ball.

2 Throw the ball to your partner and step to the right again.

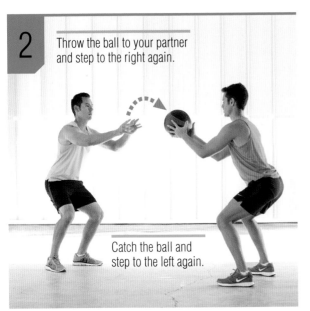

Catch the ball and step to the left again.

3 After catching the ball, step to the right again.

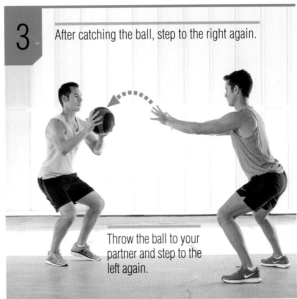

Throw the ball to your partner and step to the left again.

4 After repeating steps 2 and 3 for 5 to 10 paces in one direction, reverse your movements to return to your starting positions.

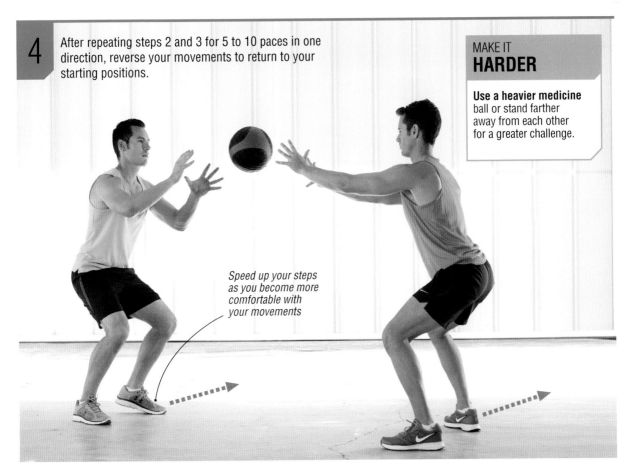

Speed up your steps as you become more comfortable with your movements

MAKE IT
HARDER

Use a heavier medicine ball or stand farther away from each other for a greater challenge.

LEVEL 2

FLOATING PLANK & SHOULDER PRESS

REQUIRED EQUIPMENT **RESISTANCE BAND**

Both partners can expect to fire up their upper bodies and cores during this exercise. Just remember that communication is key to staying in sync. You should also talk with each other as you complete each repetition to minimize overexertion and injury.

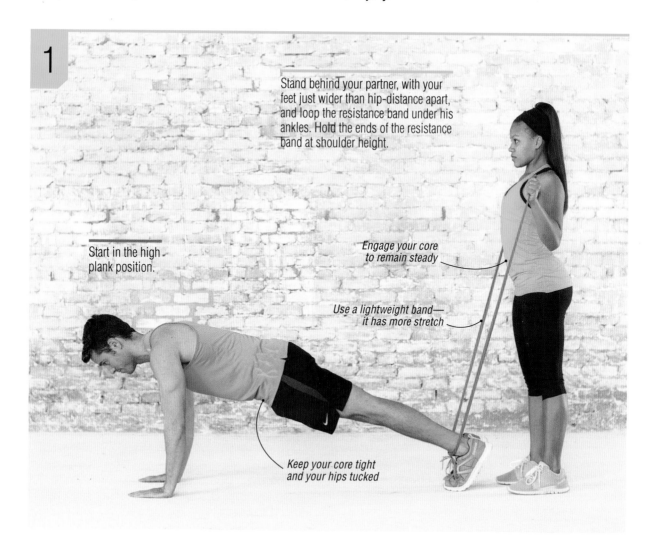

1

Stand behind your partner, with your feet just wider than hip-distance apart, and loop the resistance band under his ankles. Hold the ends of the resistance band at shoulder height.

Start in the high plank position.

Engage your core to remain steady

Use a lightweight band— it has more stretch

Keep your core tight and your hips tucked

2

Lift your arms up over your head into a shoulder press while your partner performs the hop.

Keep the resistance band as taut as you can during your partner's hop

Engage your abs and hop your feet into the air, momentarily floating in plank with the band's assistance.

Bend your knees slightly, keeping your weight in your heels for better balance

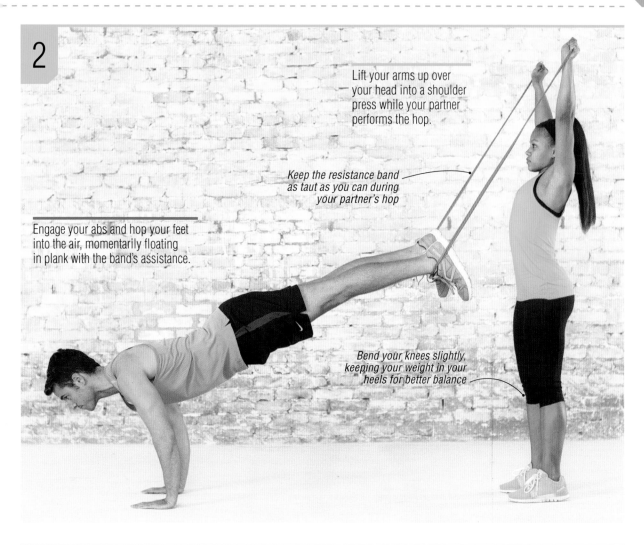

3

Reverse your shoulder press movements, bending your elbows and returning your hands to shoulder height.

Focus on keeping your lower back, hips, and abs contracted

Continue to engage your core as your feet land back down, slightly bending your knees to help reduce the impact.

MAKE IT
HARDER

Use two bands of equal resistance. Loop each one around a different ankle, holding one band in your right hand and the other in your left hand. This will allow your arms to work independently.

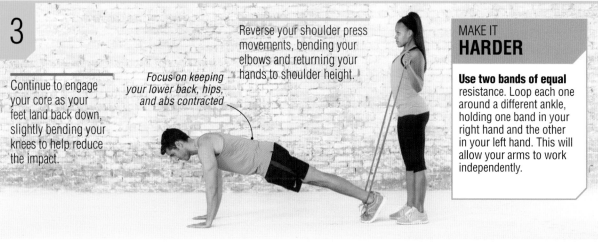

BEAR CRAWL & STATIC ROW

REQUIRED EQUIPMENT **RESISTANCE BAND**

How quickly and how intensely you perform the bear crawl portion of this exercise determines how much each partner gains from the speed and force of the movement. Expect your whole body to burn— from your calves to your abs to your shoulders.

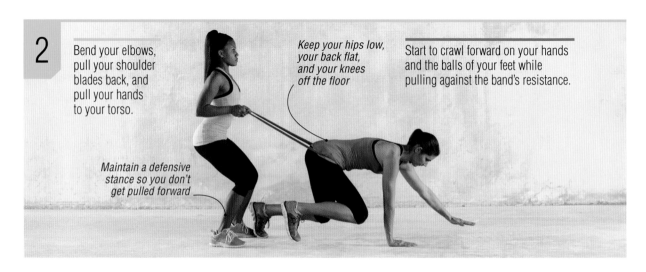

1 Stand behind your partner, with your knees bent slightly, and hold the resistance band with both hands.

The resistance band should be taut, not tight

Start on your hands and knees, with the resistance band looped around your waist.

2 Bend your elbows, pull your shoulder blades back, and pull your hands to your torso.

Keep your hips low, your back flat, and your knees off the floor

Start to crawl forward on your hands and the balls of your feet while pulling against the band's resistance.

Maintain a defensive stance so you don't get pulled forward

3

Hold your footing while your partner continues to crawl forward.

Continue to crawl forward until the resistance band is fully stretched.

When the resistance band becomes fully stretched, the partner on the floor can add mountain climbers to the movement by hopping one foot forward and then quickly switching leg positions by hopping the opposite foot forward.

Engage your core and slightly bend your knees to remain steady

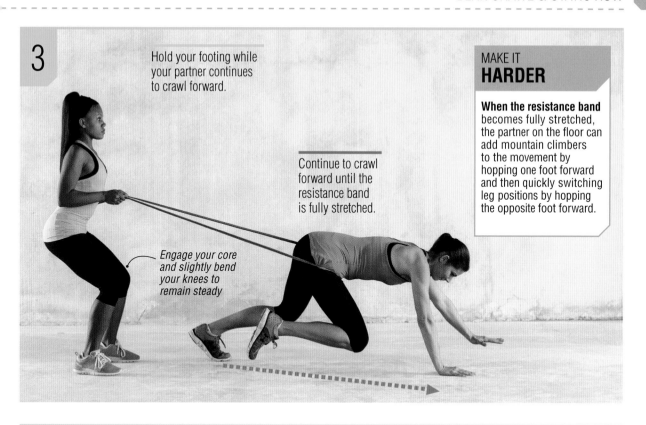

4

Repeat steps 2 through 4 for the time listed in the workout or as desired.

Maintain your position while your partner returns to her starting position.

Crawl forward and backward as fast as you can while maintaining good form

Reverse your movements to crawl backward to your starting position.

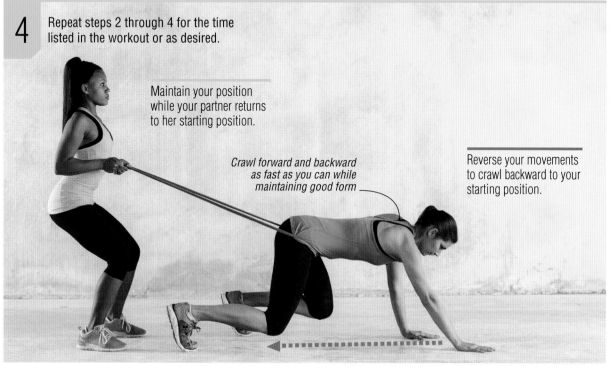

LEVEL 2

LATERAL MEDICINE BALL TOSS

REQUIRED EQUIPMENT **MEDICINE BALL**

Rotating laterally while throwing a medicine ball works your shoulders and obliques while improving your upper-body power. Start with a lightweight medicine ball to master the movements before trying this exercise with a heavier ball.

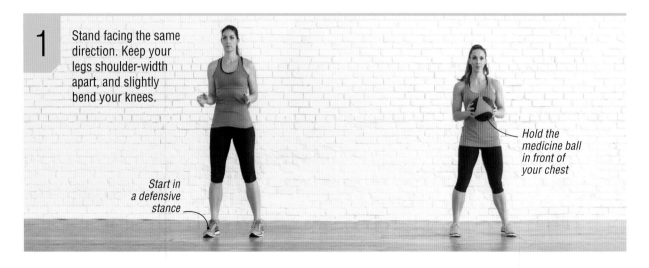

1 Stand facing the same direction. Keep your legs shoulder-width apart, and slightly bend your knees.

Start in a defensive stance

Hold the medicine ball in front of your chest

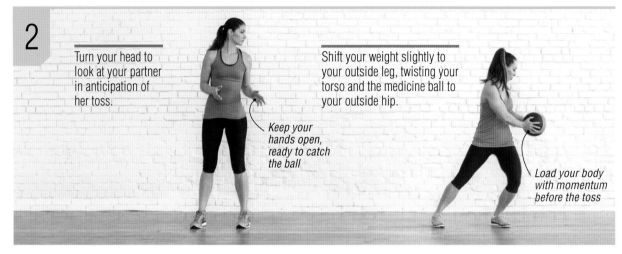

2 Turn your head to look at your partner in anticipation of her toss.

Keep your hands open, ready to catch the ball

Shift your weight slightly to your outside leg, twisting your torso and the medicine ball to your outside hip.

Load your body with momentum before the toss

3   Tighten your core to protect your back.

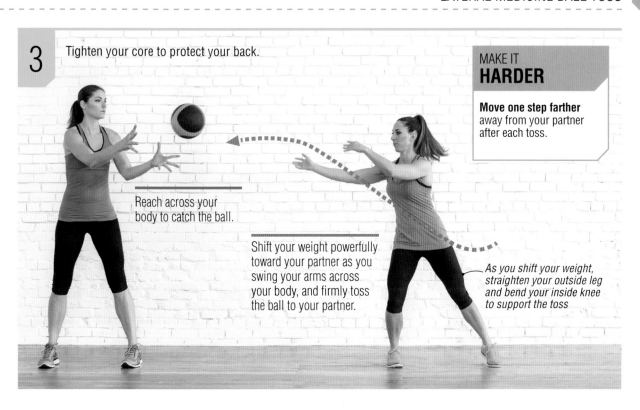

MAKE IT
HARDER

Move one step farther away from your partner after each toss.

Reach across your body to catch the ball.

Shift your weight powerfully toward your partner as you swing your arms across your body, and firmly toss the ball to your partner.

As you shift your weight, straighten your outside leg and bend your inside knee to support the toss

4   Repeat steps 2 through 4 for the time listed in the workout or as desired.

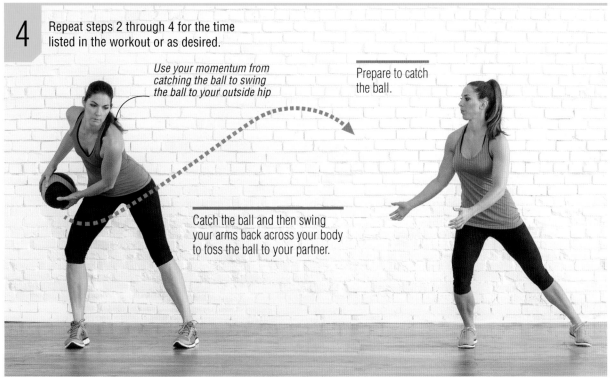

Use your momentum from catching the ball to swing the ball to your outside hip

Prepare to catch the ball.

Catch the ball and then swing your arms back across your body to toss the ball to your partner.

LEVEL 2

UNSTABLE PUSHUP & MEDICINE BALL ROLL

REQUIRED EQUIPMENT   **2 MEDICINE BALLS OF EQUAL DIAMETERS**

The balance and coordination requirements for this exercise add an extra challenge to an otherwise classic upper-body movement that targets the chest, triceps, and stabilizing muscles of the core. The balls can be any weight but should have the same diameter.

1 Start in the high plank position, facing each other, with a medicine ball under your right palms.

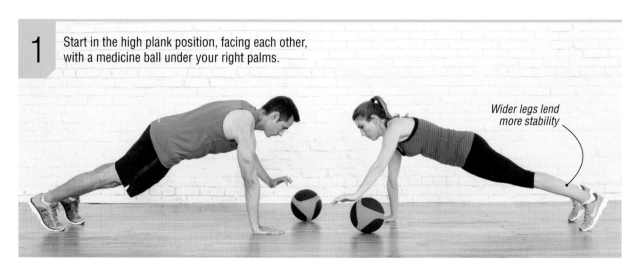

Wider legs lend more stability

2 Go down into a pushup, and as you return to—and maintain—your high plank position, roll your ball straight across to your partner.

Keep the ball positioned under your shoulder throughout your pushup

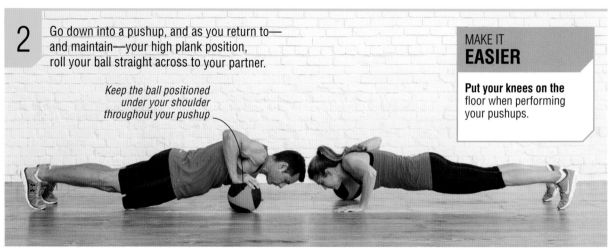

MAKE IT
EASIER

Put your knees on the floor when performing your pushups.

3 Roll your ball—now under your left palm—straight across to your partner before going down into another pushup.

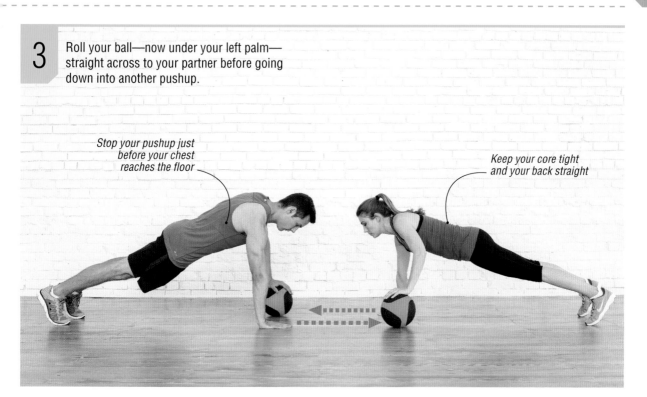

Stop your pushup just before your chest reaches the floor

Keep your core tight and your back straight

4 Raise back up into the high plank position, rolling your ball toward your partner again.

Keep your neck aligned with your spine—and avoid dropping or craning your head when you perform your pushups

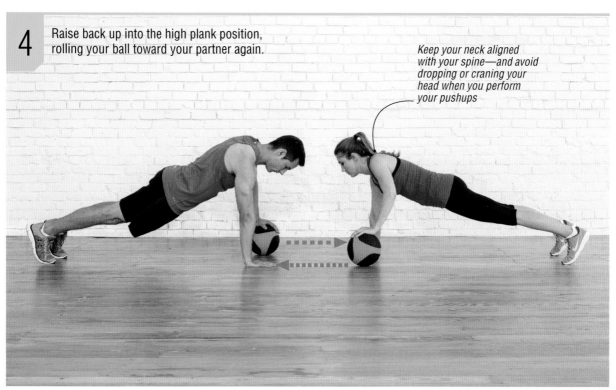

WALL SQUAT & MEDICINE BALL SITUP

REQUIRED EQUIPMENT **MEDICINE BALL**

In your different roles for this exercise, you'll work your core, your glutes, and your arms. If you move farther away from your partner, you'll also increase the workload to your upper body while throwing the medicine ball back and forth.

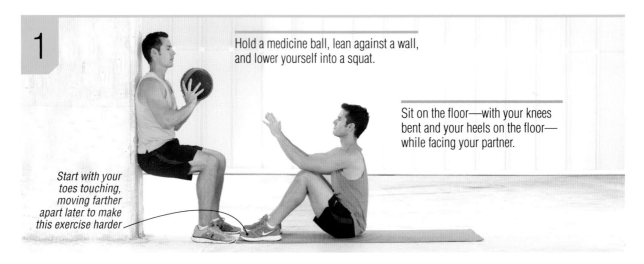

1

Hold a medicine ball, lean against a wall, and lower yourself into a squat.

Sit on the floor—with your knees bent and your heels on the floor— while facing your partner.

Start with your toes touching, moving farther apart later to make this exercise harder

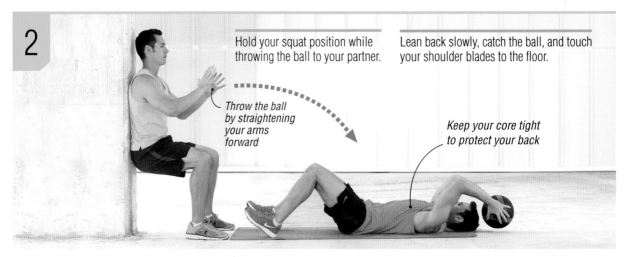

2

Hold your squat position while throwing the ball to your partner.

Lean back slowly, catch the ball, and touch your shoulder blades to the floor.

Throw the ball by straightening your arms forward

Keep your core tight to protect your back

3

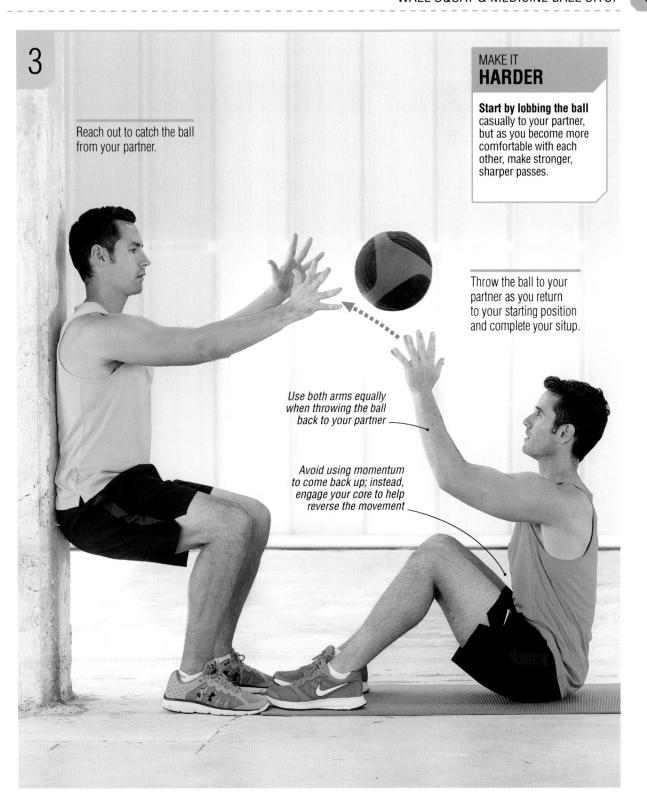

Reach out to catch the ball from your partner.

MAKE IT
HARDER

Start by lobbing the ball casually to your partner, but as you become more comfortable with each other, make stronger, sharper passes.

Throw the ball to your partner as you return to your starting position and complete your situp.

Use both arms equally when throwing the ball back to your partner

Avoid using momentum to come back up; instead, engage your core to help reverse the movement

BOSU SQUAT & RESISTANCE BAND ROW

REQUIRED EQUIPMENT **2 BOSU BALLS • 2 RESISTANCE BANDS OF EQUAL RESISTANCE**

You'll build strength in your glutes, quads, back, and core while challenging your balance and coordination with this full-body BOSU exercise. If you're new to balance exercises, make the movements easier by flipping the BOSU ball over so the dome side faces up.

1 Facing your partner, stand on a BOSU ball and hold one end of each band in each hand.

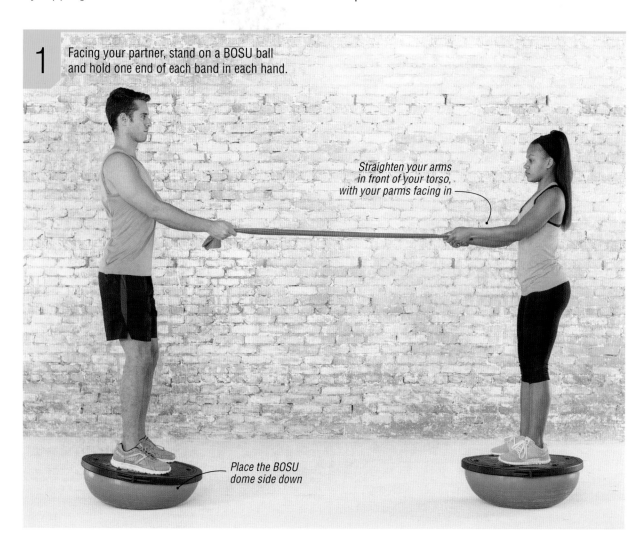

Straighten your arms in front of your torso, with your parms facing in

Place the BOSU dome side down

2 Squat down as you simultaneously pull against the resistance bands, bending your elbows and pulling your arms back.

MAKE IT
HARDER

Turn this exercise into an advanced move by doing a single-leg squat rather than a two-legged squat.

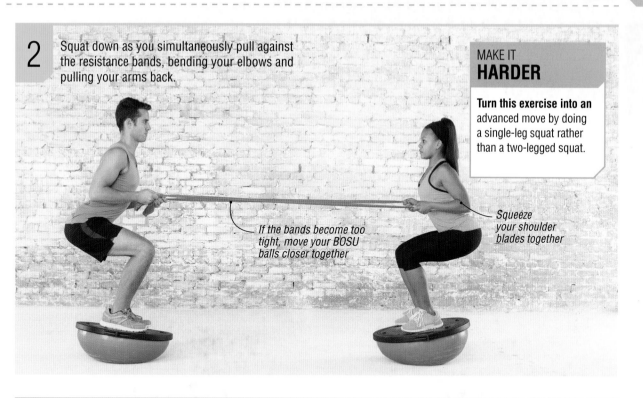

If the bands become too tight, move your BOSU balls closer together

Squeeze your shoulder blades together

3 Push through your heels, returning to standing as you straighten your arms to their original position.

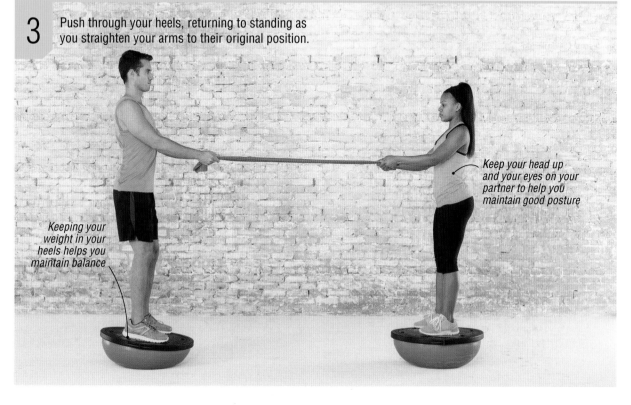

Keeping your weight in your heels helps you maintain balance

Keep your head up and your eyes on your partner to help you maintain good posture

WALL SQUAT & OVERHEAD DUMBBELL SHOULDER PRESS

REQUIRED EQUIPMENT **DUMBBELLS**

During this up close and personal partner move, the partner in the wall squat acts as a chair for the partner performing the shoulder press, whose weight makes the wall squat more challenging. After doing both positions, you'll have enjoyed a full-body workout.

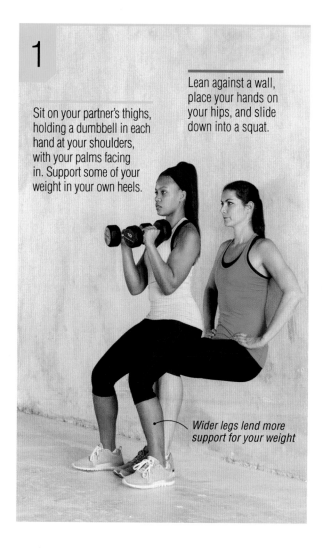

1

Lean against a wall, place your hands on your hips, and slide down into a squat.

Sit on your partner's thighs, holding a dumbbell in each hand at your shoulders, with your palms facing in. Support some of your weight in your own heels.

Wider legs lend more support for your weight

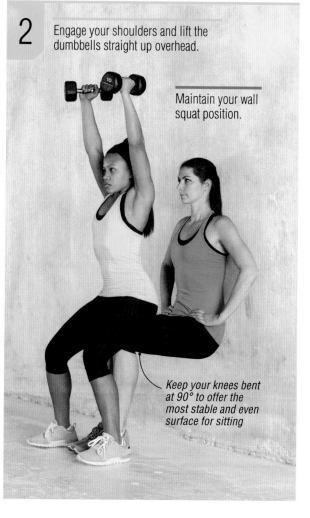

2

Engage your shoulders and lift the dumbbells straight up overhead.

Maintain your wall squat position.

Keep your knees bent at 90° to offer the most stable and even surface for sitting

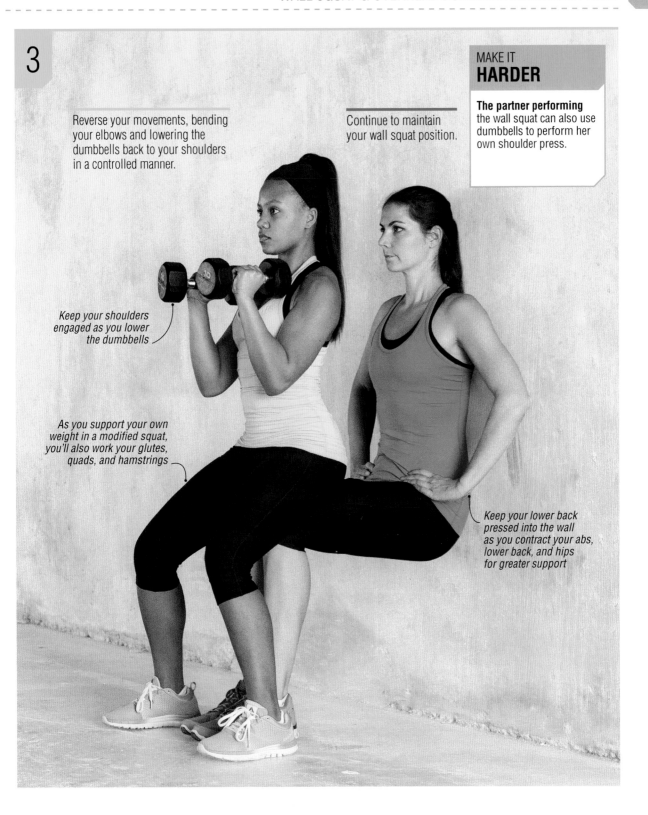

3

Reverse your movements, bending your elbows and lowering the dumbbells back to your shoulders in a controlled manner.

Continue to maintain your wall squat position.

MAKE IT
HARDER

The partner performing the wall squat can also use dumbbells to perform her own shoulder press.

Keep your shoulders engaged as you lower the dumbbells

As you support your own weight in a modified squat, you'll also work your glutes, quads, and hamstrings

Keep your lower back pressed into the wall as you contract your abs, lower back, and hips for greater support

LEVEL 2

LEG THROWS

REQUIRED EQUIPMENT   **NONE**

Mix up your everyday abdominal routine with this exercise. The partner performing the leg lift challenges her abs by working against her partner's throws, while the other partner enjoys a chest and arm workout for upper-body power.

1

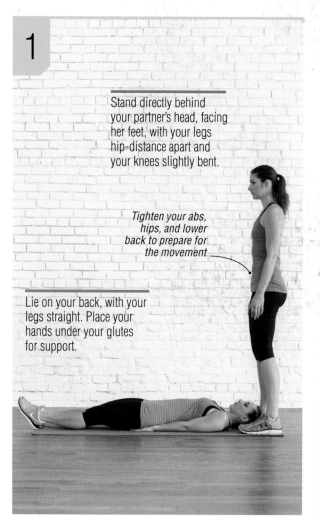

Stand directly behind your partner's head, facing her feet, with your legs hip-distance apart and your knees slightly bent.

Tighten your abs, hips, and lower back to prepare for the movement

Lie on your back, with your legs straight. Place your hands under your glutes for support.

2

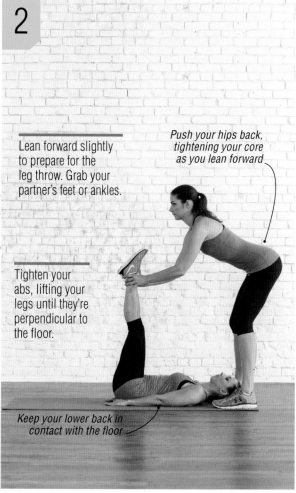

Lean forward slightly to prepare for the leg throw. Grab your partner's feet or ankles.

Push your hips back, tightening your core as you lean forward

Tighten your abs, lifting your legs until they're perpendicular to the floor.

Keep your lower back in contact with the floor

3

Forcefully throw your partner's feet or ankles toward the floor.

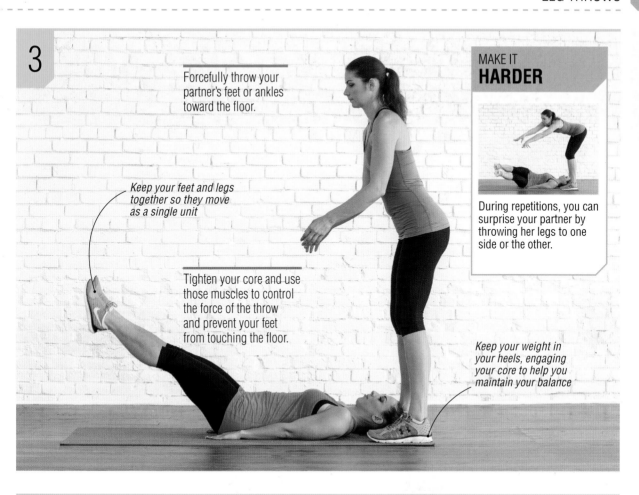

Keep your feet and legs together so they move as a single unit

During repetitions, you can surprise your partner by throwing her legs to one side or the other.

Tighten your core and use those muscles to control the force of the throw and prevent your feet from touching the floor.

Keep your weight in your heels, engaging your core to help you maintain your balance

4

Perform steps 2 through 4 for the time or reps listed in the workout or as desired.

Straighten back up, preparing for the next throw.

Raise your feet up again.

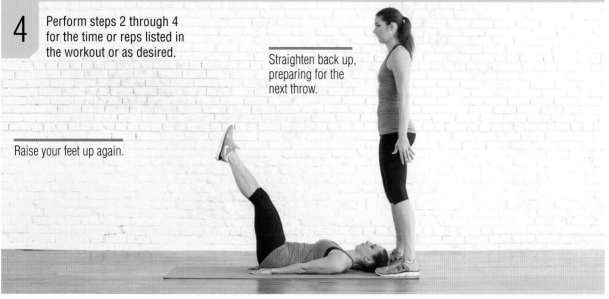

POWER PLANK & CHEST PRESS

REQUIRED EQUIPMENT **STABILITY BALL • BOSU BALL**

This exercise works your chest, triceps, shoulders, abs, and hips. It's an advanced movement, and it's not for those shy about intensity. Before trying this exercise, you should have mastered the jumping and balance exercises in levels 1 and 2.

1

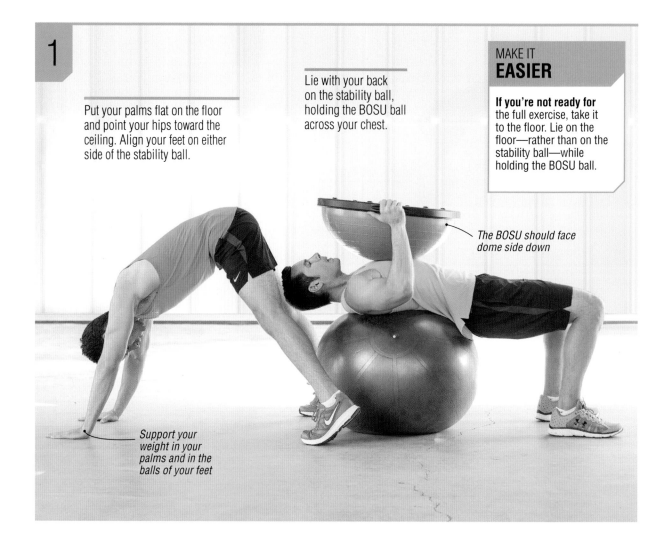

Put your palms flat on the floor and point your hips toward the ceiling. Align your feet on either side of the stability ball.

Lie with your back on the stability ball, holding the BOSU ball across your chest.

The BOSU should face dome side down

Support your weight in your palms and in the balls of your feet

MAKE IT EASIER

If you're not ready for the full exercise, take it to the floor. Lie on the floor—rather than on the stability ball—while holding the BOSU ball.

2

Hold the BOSU steady, anticipating your partner's motions.

Push through your palms as you jump your feet up and in, landing them on the BOSU.

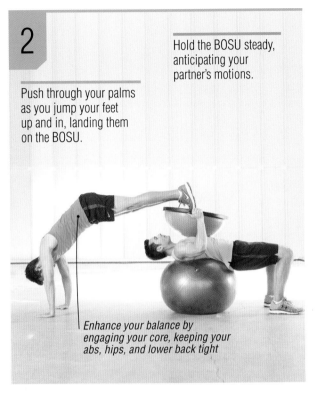

Enhance your balance by engaging your core, keeping your abs, hips, and lower back tight

3

Perform a chest press by straightening your elbows to lift the BOSU away from your chest. Keep the BOSU steady to help your partner maintain his balance.

Hold your position while your partner performs a chest press.

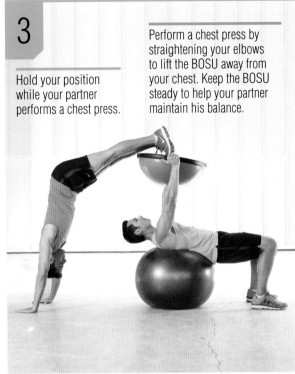

4

Carefully lower the BOSU back to your chest.

Maintain your position while your partner lowers the BOSU.

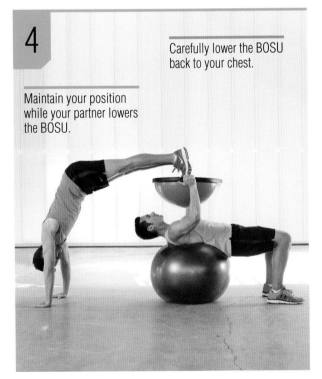

5

Hop your feet back to the floor on each side of the stability ball.

Continue to hold the BOSU steady while your partner jumps off the BOSU.

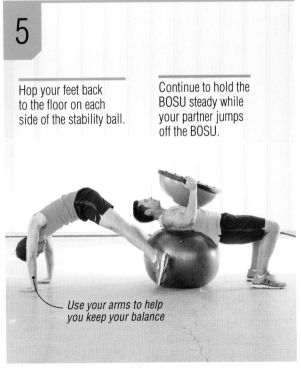

Use your arms to help you keep your balance

BOSU PUSHUP & SHOULDER SQUAT

REQUIRED EQUIPMENT **BOSU BALL**

The positions for this full-body exercise are challenging, but if you can manage the initial setup, you can manage this exercise. Pay close attention to proper squat and pushup form to maximize this exercise's challenge while minimizing the risk of injury.

1

To get into position, begin by squatting low at your partner's feet. As your partner lifts one leg at a time, help him position each foot over your corresponding shoulder. Return to standing.

Start in the high plank position, placing your hands on the inverted BOSU. When your partner's ready, lift one leg at a time to hook your feet over her shoulders, keeping your core tight and straight.

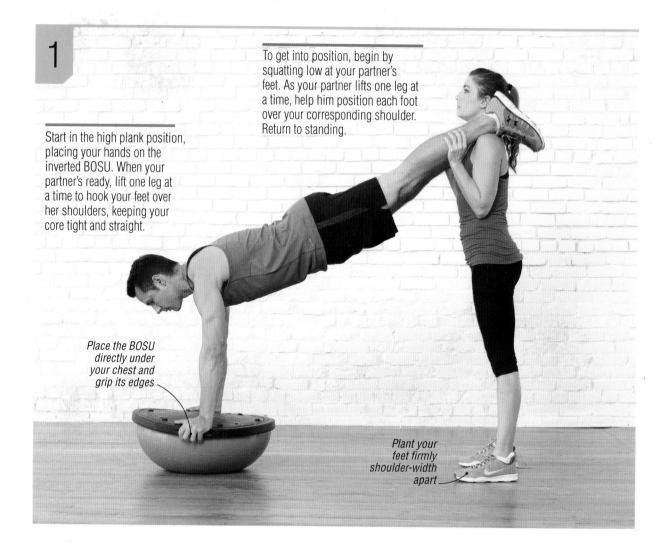

Place the BOSU directly under your chest and grip its edges

Plant your feet firmly shoulder-width apart

2

Holding your partner's ankles at your shoulders, bend your knees and sit back into a squat.

Push your hips back, and look up slightly to keep your chest lifted

Bend your elbows and perform a pushup as you lower your chest toward the BOSU.

The lowest point of the pushup is when your elbows are at or just below 90°

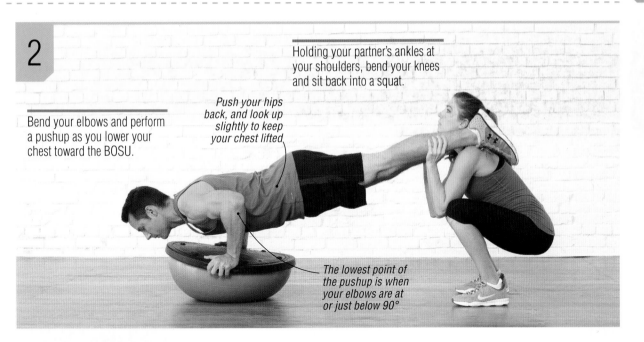

3

Push through your heels, straightening your knees and hips to return to standing.

Push through your palms, straightening your elbows to push yourself back to your original high plank position.

Align your shoulders with your palms when you return to the high plank position

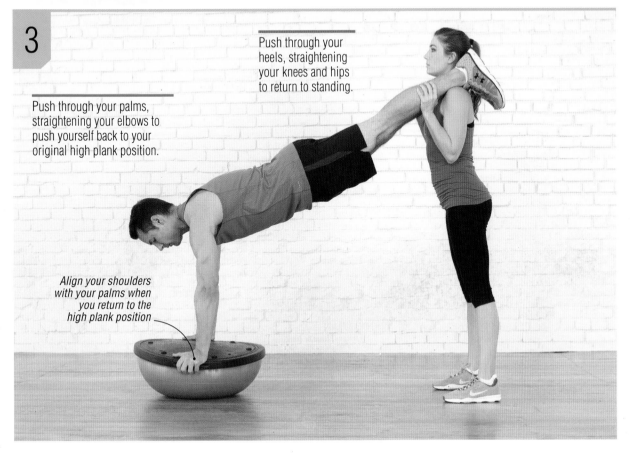

STABILITY BALL REVERSE CURL & TRICEPS ROLLOUT

REQUIRED EQUIPMENT **STABILITY BALL**

This fun exercise is bound to generate a few laughs as you master the move because you might tumble off the ball at first; don't be surprised if it takes a few attempts. Both partners will receive a great core workout, targeting the abs, hips, lower back, and shoulder girdle.

1

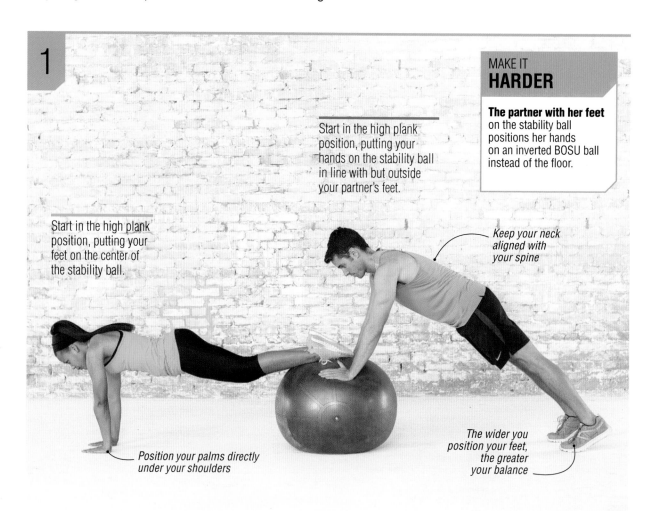

Start in the high plank position, putting your hands on the stability ball in line with but outside your partner's feet.

Start in the high plank position, putting your feet on the center of the stability ball.

Position your palms directly under your shoulders

Keep your neck aligned with your spine

The wider you position your feet, the greater your balance

MAKE IT HARDER

The partner with her feet on the stability ball positions her hands on an inverted BOSU ball instead of the floor.

2

Engage your core, pulling your knees toward your chest while using your feet to pull the ball toward you.

As the ball rolls away from you, bend your elbows, allowing your palms to roll forward until your forearms are on the ball.

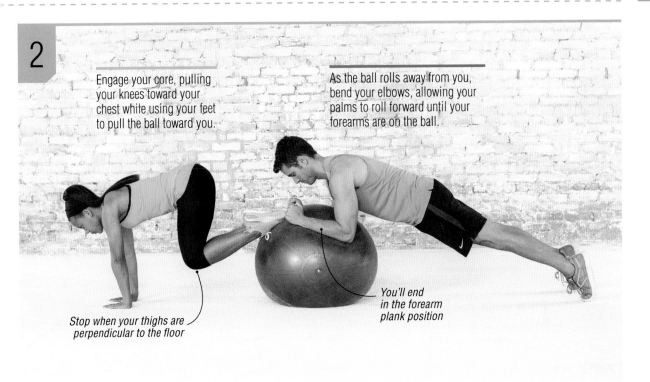

Stop when your thighs are perpendicular to the floor

You'll end in the forearm plank position

3

Perform steps 2 and 3 for the time listed in the workout or as desired.

Return to your high plank position by using your triceps to push through your palms, straightening your elbows as the ball rolls toward you.

Reverse your movements, pushing your feet away from you as you return to the high plank position.

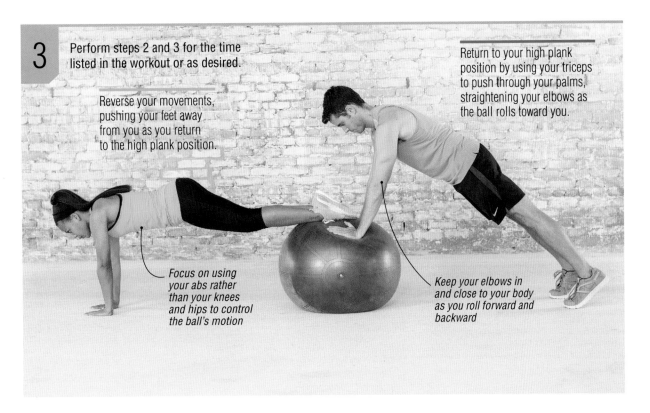

Focus on using your abs rather than your knees and hips to control the ball's motion

Keep your elbows in and close to your body as you roll forward and backward

COORDINATED STABILITY BALL HAMSTRING CURLS

REQUIRED EQUIPMENT **STABILITY BALL**

The backs of your thighs will scream by the end of this exercise because you'll use them to keep your glutes and hips off the floor. The resistance comes from your own body weight as well as gravity, while the stability ball incorporates an added balance challenge.

1

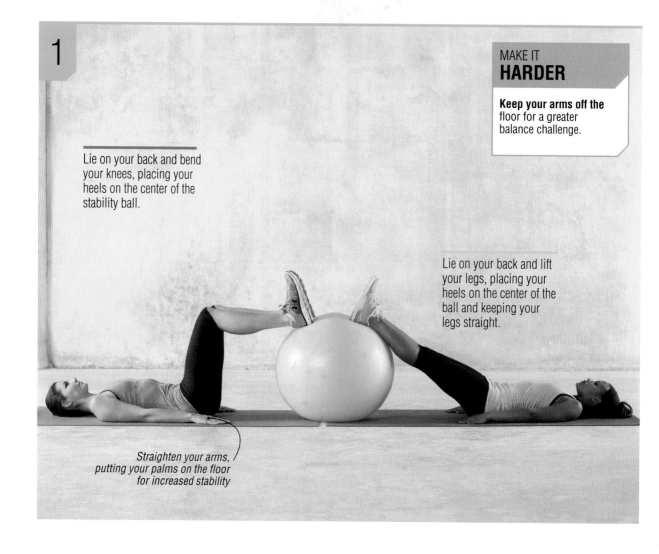

MAKE IT
HARDER

Keep your arms off the floor for a greater balance challenge.

Lie on your back and bend your knees, placing your heels on the center of the stability ball.

Lie on your back and lift your legs, placing your heels on the center of the ball and keeping your legs straight.

Straighten your arms, putting your palms on the floor for increased stability

2

Lift your hips off the floor to form a bent-knee bridge.

Press your heels firmly into the ball to help you enter the bridge position

Tighten your glutes, raising your hips off the floor to form a straight-leg bridge.

Keep your glutes and thighs off the floor throughout

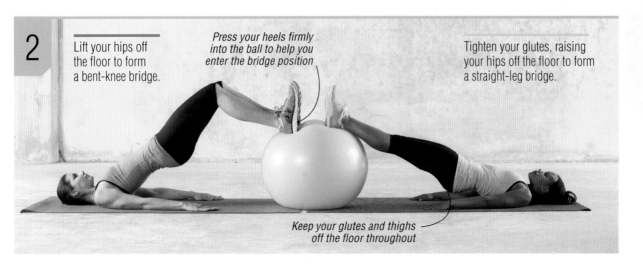

3

Maintaining a strong core and keeping your hips up, straighten your legs, using your heels to push the stability ball away from you.

Tighten your core, lifting your hips higher as you bend your knees, and use your heels to pull the stability ball toward you.

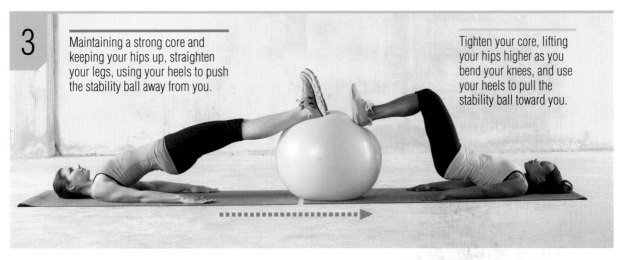

4

Perform steps 2 through 4 for the time listed in the workout or as desired.

Straighten your legs as you push the stability ball away from your body.

Bend your knees to pull the stability ball back toward you.

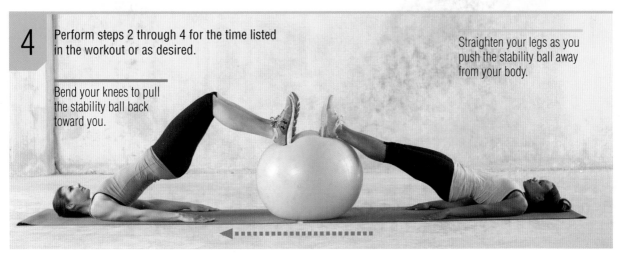

COORDINATED STABILITY BALL LUNGES

REQUIRED EQUIPMENT **STABILITY BALL**

This exercise will target your entire lower body—hamstrings, quads, glutes, and even calves—while also requiring balance, coordination, and a lot of communication. Pay close attention to the starting positions to ensure you sync up correctly with your partner.

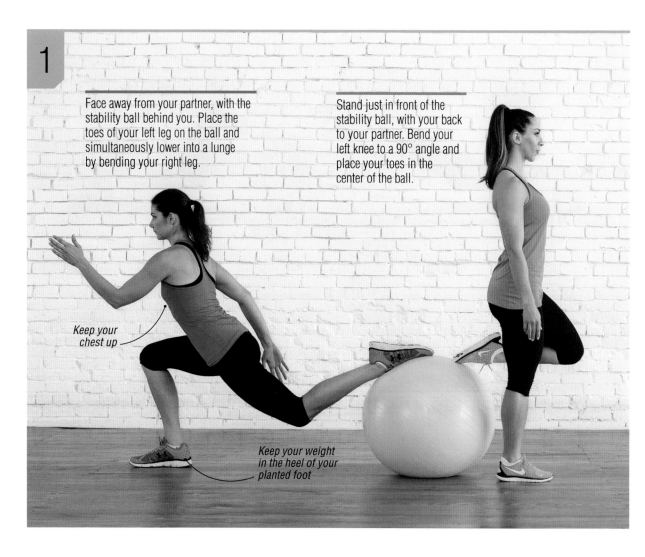

1

Face away from your partner, with the stability ball behind you. Place the toes of your left leg on the ball and simultaneously lower into a lunge by bending your right leg.

Stand just in front of the stability ball, with your back to your partner. Bend your left knee to a 90° angle and place your toes in the center of the ball.

Keep your chest up

Keep your weight in the heel of your planted foot

2

Press through your right heel, using your left foot to pull the ball toward your body as you rise to standing.

Press through the ball with your toes, straightening your left leg as you bend your right knee to lower yourself into a lunge.

Roll the ball with your foot

Use your arms for balance by swinging your left arm forward as you push the ball away with your left foot

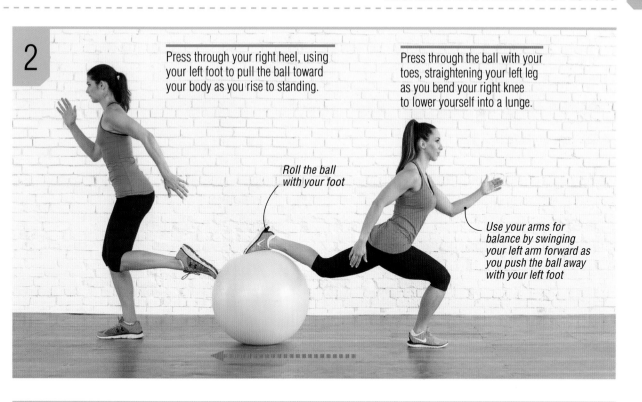

3

Perform steps 2 through 3 for the time listed in the workout or as desired.

Bend your right knee, lowering your hips as you straighten your left leg behind you and return to your starting position.

Use your foot to help pull the ball back toward you as you push through your front heel and return to your starting position.

VARIATION

Stand on opposite sides of the ball, facing the wall, with your inside legs positioned atop the ball. One partner performs a side lunge while the other stands with a bent knee. Alternate the lunges.

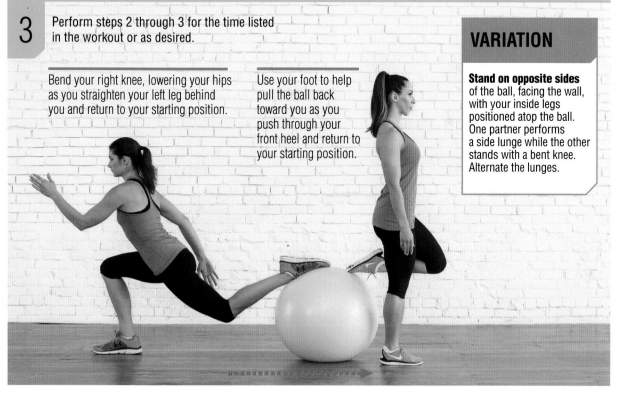

WEIGHTED PLANK & DUMBBELL CHEST PRESS

REQUIRED EQUIPMENT   **2 DUMBBELLS**

Getting into position for the plank and chest press might feel a little awkward, which is why it's an advanced move. Tightening your glutes, hips, abdominals, back, chest, and shoulders is critical, particularly to help support your partner's weight when you're performing the plank.

1

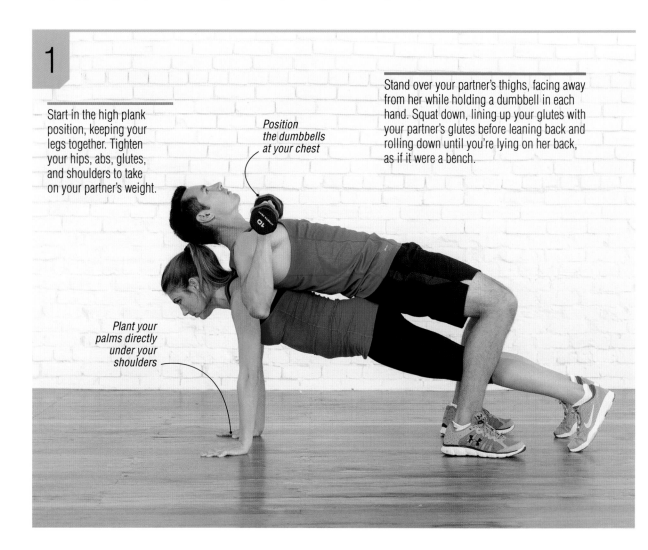

Start in the high plank position, keeping your legs together. Tighten your hips, abs, glutes, and shoulders to take on your partner's weight.

Position the dumbbells at your chest

Stand over your partner's thighs, facing away from her while holding a dumbbell in each hand. Squat down, lining up your glutes with your partner's glutes before leaning back and rolling down until you're lying on her back, as if it were a bench.

Plant your palms directly under your shoulders

2

Maintain your high plank position, spreading your feet wider if necessary to provide a broader base of support.

Push through your heels and up through your hips for additional support. Straighten your elbows, pushing the dumbbells straight up over your chest.

MAKE IT
HARDER

Use heavier dumbbells. The added weight—and having to support it—will make this exercise more challenging for both partners.

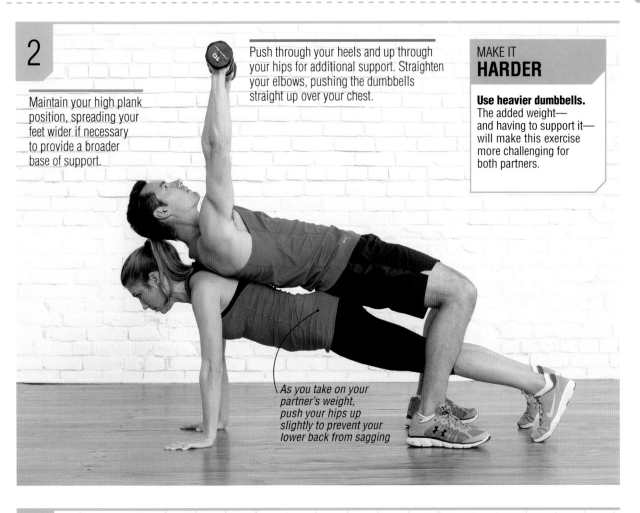

As you take on your partner's weight, push your hips up slightly to prevent your lower back from sagging

3

Perform steps 2 and 3 for the time listed in the workout or as desired.

Reverse your movements, bending your elbows and lowering the dumbbells to your chest in a controlled manner.

Continue to maintain your high plank position.

Maintaining the high plank while supporting your partner is hard—let him know if you need a break

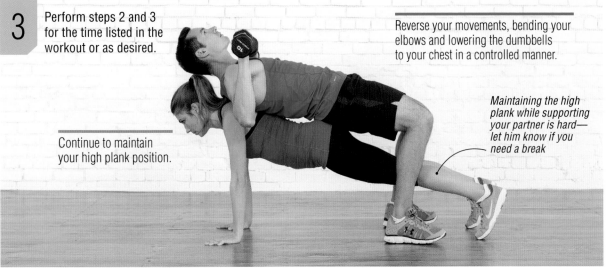

STABILITY BALL SITUP & MEDICINE BALL PASS

REQUIRED EQUIPMENT **STABILITY BALL • MEDICINE BALL**

This exercise isn't your average abdominal exercise. Catching and throwing a medicine ball while performing a situp on a stability ball requires balance, coordination, core strength, and upper-body power. You'll work your hip flexors and abs as well as your chest and triceps.

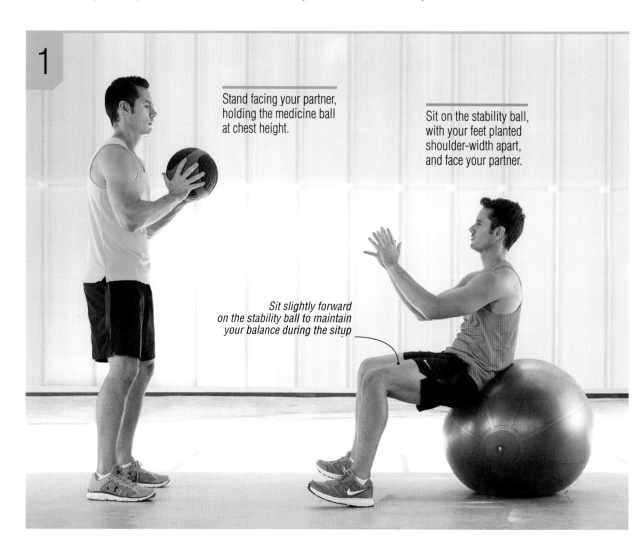

1

Stand facing your partner, holding the medicine ball at chest height.

Sit on the stability ball, with your feet planted shoulder-width apart, and face your partner.

Sit slightly forward on the stability ball to maintain your balance during the situp

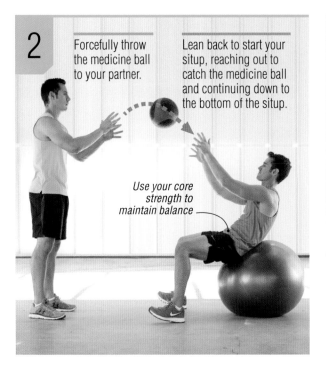

2 Forcefully throw the medicine ball to your partner.

Lean back to start your situp, reaching out to catch the medicine ball and continuing down to the bottom of the situp.

Use your core strength to maintain balance

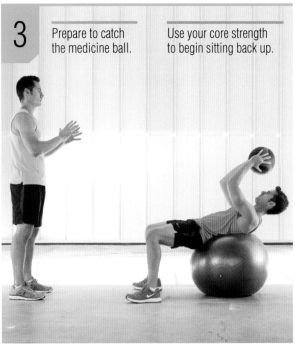

3 Prepare to catch the medicine ball.

Use your core strength to begin sitting back up.

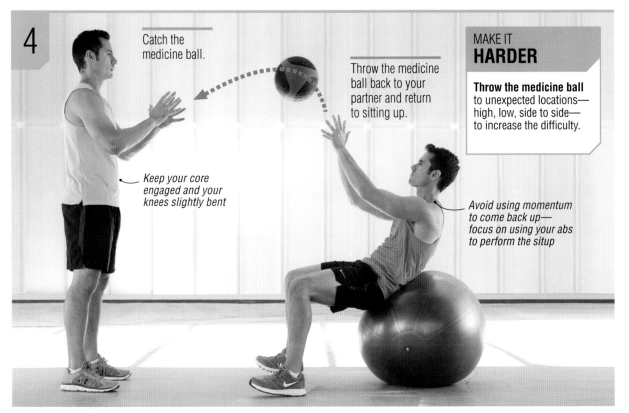

4 Catch the medicine ball.

Throw the medicine ball back to your partner and return to sitting up.

Keep your core engaged and your knees slightly bent

MAKE IT
HARDER

Throw the medicine ball to unexpected locations—high, low, side to side—to increase the difficulty.

Avoid using momentum to come back up—focus on using your abs to perform the situp

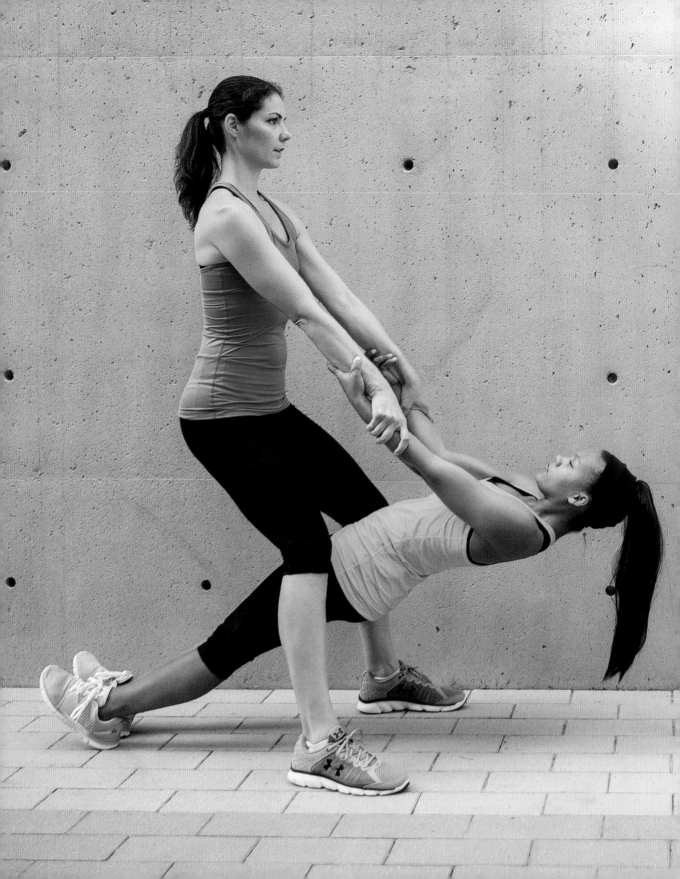

3
ASSISTED PAIRINGS EXERCISES

These exercises offer a little bit of everything: strength training, balance, coordination, cardiovascular work, and a whole lot of teamwork. What sets assisted pairings apart from other kinds of exercises is that you'll use your partner's body and your own body weight to test your physical limits.

LEVEL 1

BACK-TO-BACK SQUATS

REQUIRED EQUIPMENT **NONE**

Both partners will enjoy a total lower-body workout, including glutes, quads, calves, and hamstrings, with this exercise. The trick to properly performing the squat is for each partner to actively press against the other's back as he or she lowers his or her hips toward the floor.

1 Stand back to back with your partner, and step your feet forward once your backs are pressed together.

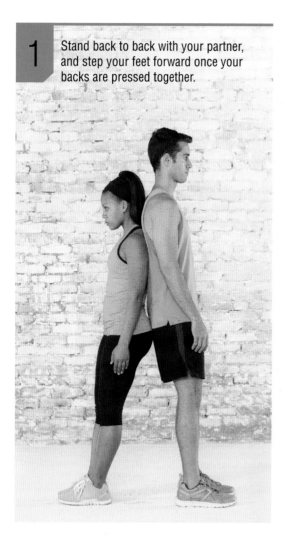

2 With your weight in your heels, bend your knees, pressing into your partner for support as you lower your hips toward the floor.

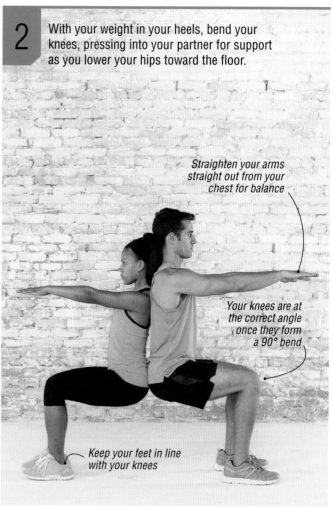

Straighten your arms straight out from your chest for balance

Your knees are at the correct angle once they form a 90° bend

Keep your feet in line with your knees

3 Push through your heels and press against your partner's back to return to standing as a single unit. Repeat steps 2 and 3 for the time listed in the workout or as desired.

VARIATION

Lower into a back-to-back squat. Twist to the left while your partner twists to the right, passing a medicine ball to your partner. Twist to the opposite side, passing the ball again. Pass the ball 10 times in each direction.

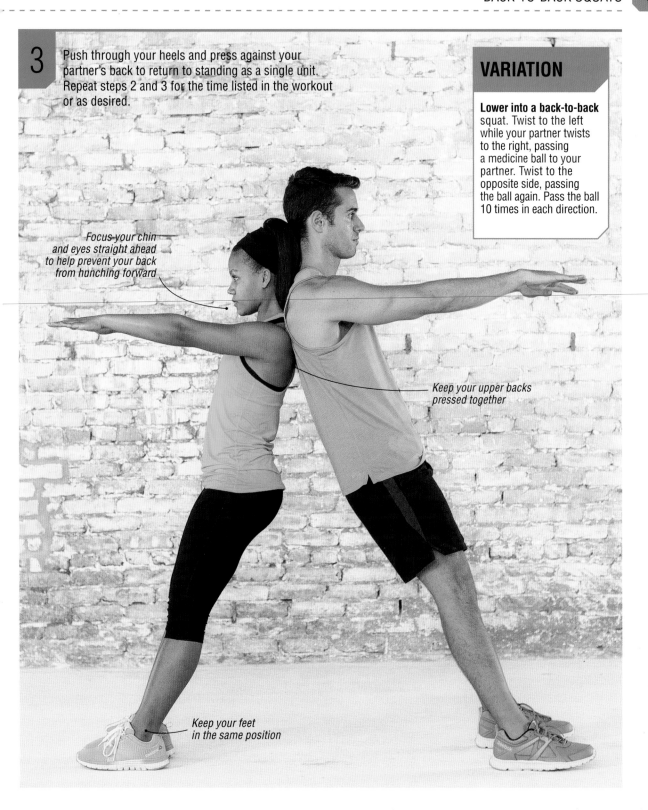

Focus your chin and eyes straight ahead to help prevent your back from hunching forward

Keep your upper backs pressed together

Keep your feet in the same position

RESISTED SHOULDER PRESS

REQUIRED EQUIPMENT **NONE**

This simple shoulder exercise is a great option when you don't have dumbbells or weights available. Plus, while the shoulder work is aimed at a specific partner, the other partner remains engaged throughout by providing the added resistance.

1

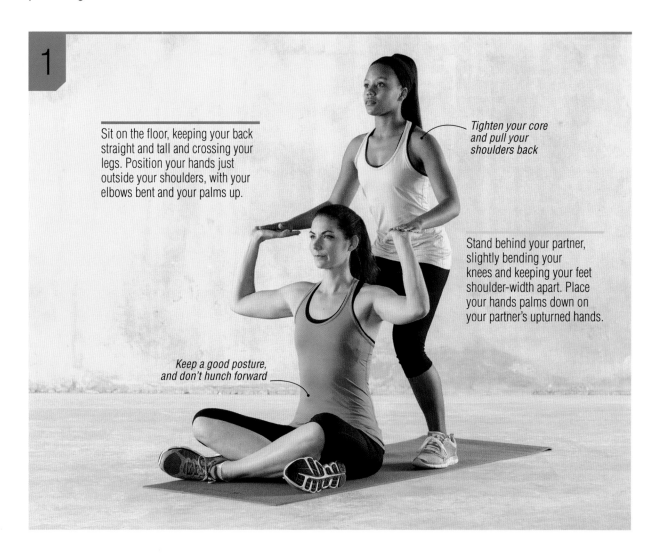

Sit on the floor, keeping your back straight and tall and crossing your legs. Position your hands just outside your shoulders, with your elbows bent and your palms up.

Tighten your core and pull your shoulders back

Stand behind your partner, slightly bending your knees and keeping your feet shoulder-width apart. Place your hands palms down on your partner's upturned hands.

Keep a good posture, and don't hunch forward

2

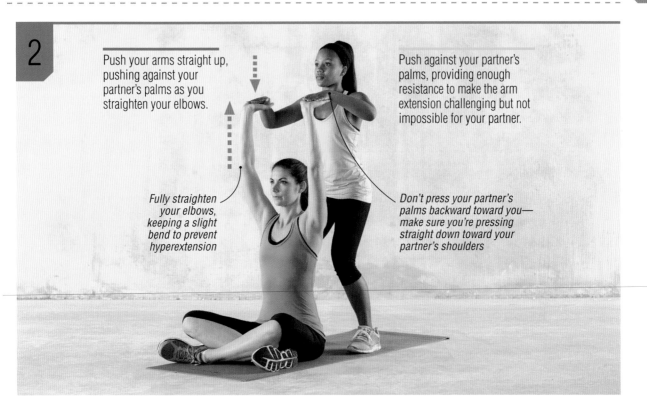

Push your arms straight up, pushing against your partner's palms as you straighten your elbows.

Fully straighten your elbows, keeping a slight bend to prevent hyperextension

Push against your partner's palms, providing enough resistance to make the arm extension challenging but not impossible for your partner.

Don't press your partner's palms backward toward you—make sure you're pressing straight down toward your partner's shoulders

3

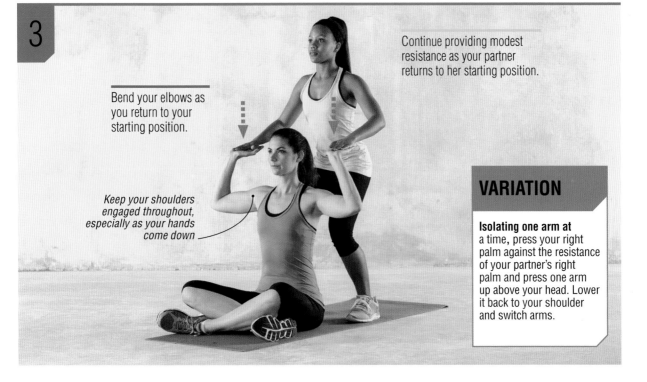

Bend your elbows as you return to your starting position.

Keep your shoulders engaged throughout, especially as your hands come down

Continue providing modest resistance as your partner returns to her starting position.

VARIATION

Isolating one arm at a time, press your right palm against the resistance of your partner's right palm and press one arm up above your head. Lower it back to your shoulder and switch arms.

LEVEL 1

COORDINATED LUNGES

REQUIRED EQUIPMENT **NONE**

These are an excellent way to increase strength in your lower body—glutes, quads, hamstrings, and calves—as you also improve balance and coordination. Remember that the same leg remains fixed throughout the exercise, while the other leg initiates each lunge.

1 Face your partner, holding each other's wrists. Your knees should be slightly bent, with your feet hip-distance apart.

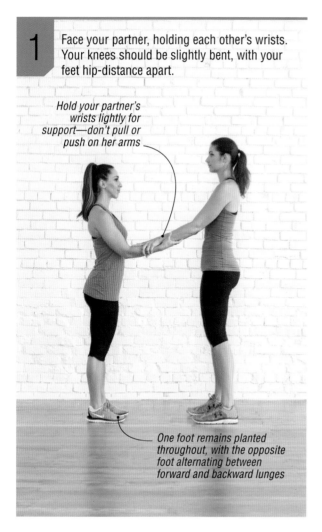

Hold your partner's wrists lightly for support—don't pull or push on her arms

One foot remains planted throughout, with the opposite foot alternating between forward and backward lunges

2

Lunge back with your left leg, planting the ball of your foot. Bend both knees, and keeping your torso tall, lower your back knee toward the floor.

Lunge forward with your right foot, planting it in front of you, with your weight in your heel. Bend both knees, lowering your back knee toward the floor.

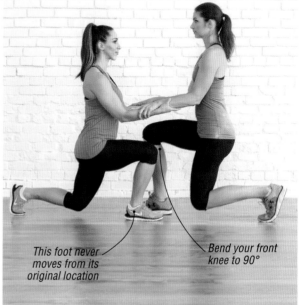

This foot never moves from its original location

Bend your front knee to 90°

3

Continue lunging forward and backward—always initiating the lunge with the same leg while your opposite foot remains stationary—for the time listed in the workout or as desired.

Coordinating the movement with your partner, press off the ball of your left foot and through the heel of your right foot, lunging your back leg forward and past your front foot. Plant your heel and lower into a lunge.

As your partner begins her second lunge, press through the heel of your right foot to return to standing. Immediately lunge your right foot backward, planting the ball of your foot before lowering into a lunge.

MAKE IT
EASIER

Rather than lunging continuously forward and backward using the same leg for each lunge, one partner will lunge backward on her left leg while the other partner lunges forward on her right leg. Both partners will return to standing before switching legs.

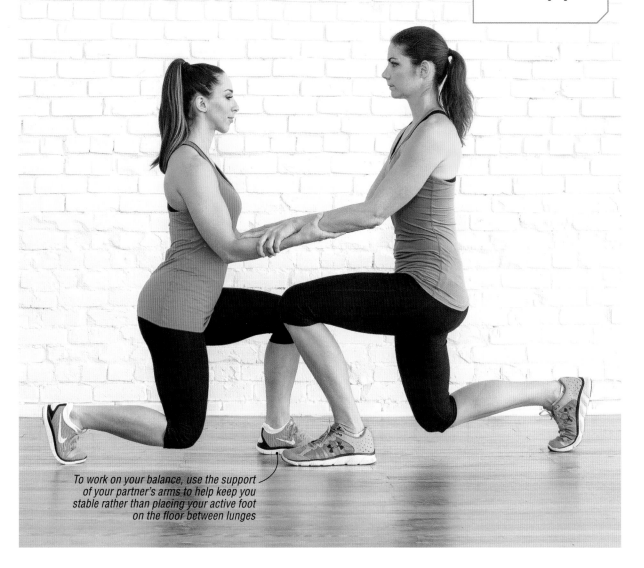

To work on your balance, use the support of your partner's arms to help keep you stable rather than placing your active foot on the floor between lunges

LEVEL 2

WALL SQUAT & DIP

REQUIRED EQUIPMENT   **NONE**

The partner holding the static wall squat will enjoy a lower-body endurance challenge, while the other partner strengthens her triceps with a bodyweight-driven dip. This exercise is perfect for circuit workouts because you can switch positions without much rest.

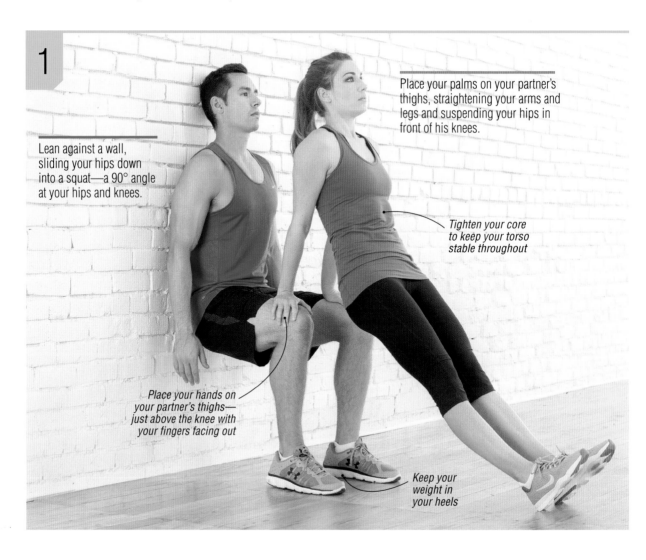

1

Place your palms on your partner's thighs, straightening your arms and legs and suspending your hips in front of his knees.

Lean against a wall, sliding your hips down into a squat—a 90° angle at your hips and knees.

Tighten your core to keep your torso stable throughout

Place your hands on your partner's thighs— just above the knee with your fingers facing out

Keep your weight in your heels

2

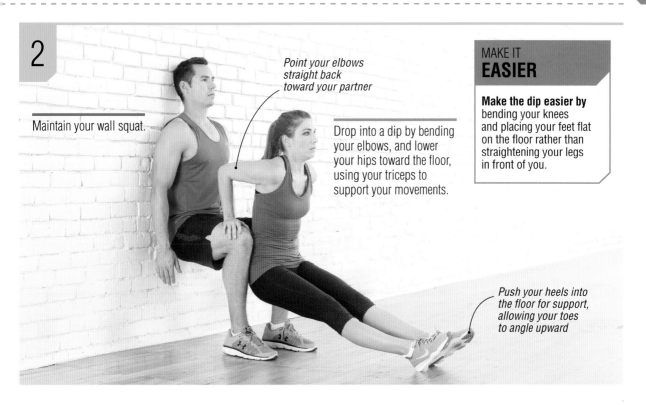

Point your elbows straight back toward your partner

Maintain your wall squat.

Drop into a dip by bending your elbows, and lower your hips toward the floor, using your triceps to support your movements.

Push your heels into the floor for support, allowing your toes to angle upward

3

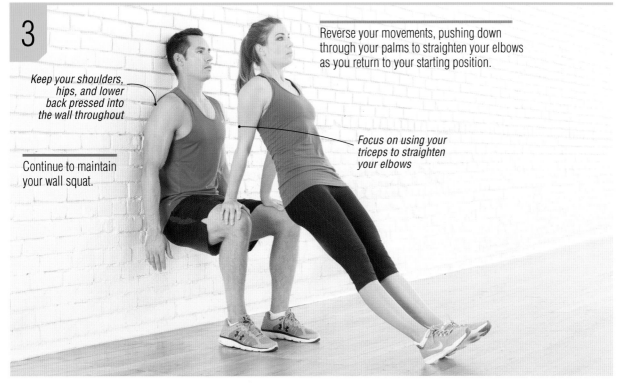

Reverse your movements, pushing down through your palms to straighten your elbows as you return to your starting position.

Keep your shoulders, hips, and lower back pressed into the wall throughout

Focus on using your triceps to straighten your elbows

Continue to maintain your wall squat.

WHEELBARROW WALK

REQUIRED EQUIPMENT **NONE**

This wheelbarrow walk might remind you of recess when you were a kid. That's a good thing because it proves that fun and games can also be exercise. This movement offers a cardio challenge for both partners, while one partner enjoys an extra dose of upper-body-strength work.

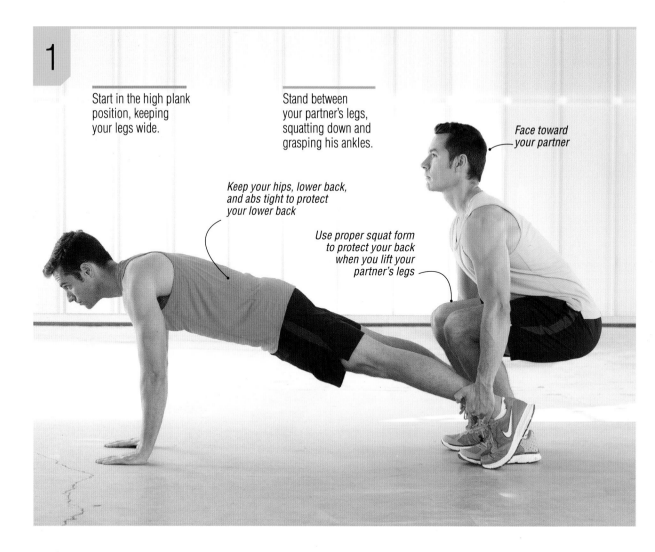

1

Start in the high plank position, keeping your legs wide.

Stand between your partner's legs, squatting down and grasping his ankles.

Face toward your partner

Keep your hips, lower back, and abs tight to protect your lower back

Use proper squat form to protect your back when you lift your partner's legs

2

Push through your heels and return to standing, lifting your partner's legs off the floor.

Tighten your core to keep your body straight as your partner lifts your legs off the floor.

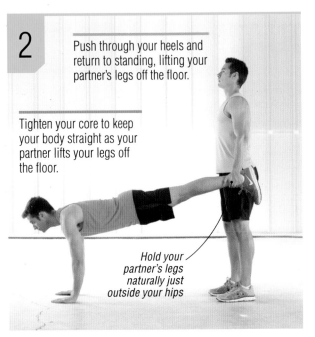

Hold your partner's legs naturally just outside your hips

3

Take a comfortable step forward with your right foot—a step that's not too long or too short.

Step your right hand forward, planting your palm.

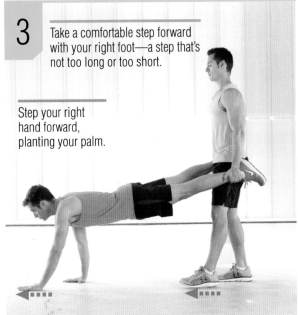

4

Repeat steps 3 and 4 for the time listed in the workout or as desired.

Step forward with your left foot—again using a normal step.

Step your left palm forward, reaching it past your right palm before planting it on the floor. Continue this right–left action with your arms.

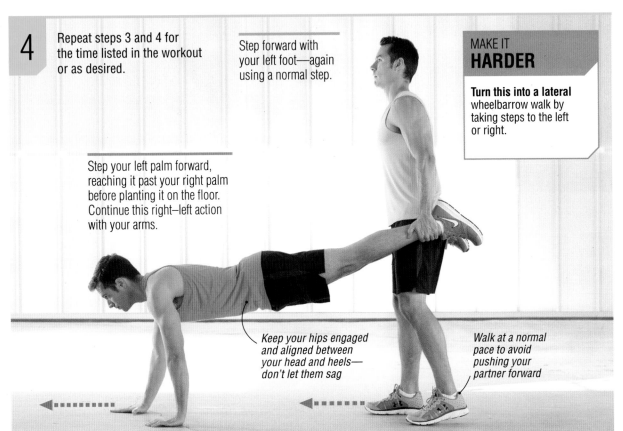

MAKE IT
HARDER

Turn this into a lateral wheelbarrow walk by taking steps to the left or right.

Keep your hips engaged and aligned between your head and heels— don't let them sag

Walk at a normal pace to avoid pushing your partner forward

WHEELBARROW SQUAT & PUSHUP

REQUIRED EQUIPMENT **NONE**

Bodyweight exercises offer an extra challenge when performed with a partner. Suspended pushups give you a great core workout, and the squat becomes weighted when you hold your partner's legs. Paired together, you'll work practically every major muscle group.

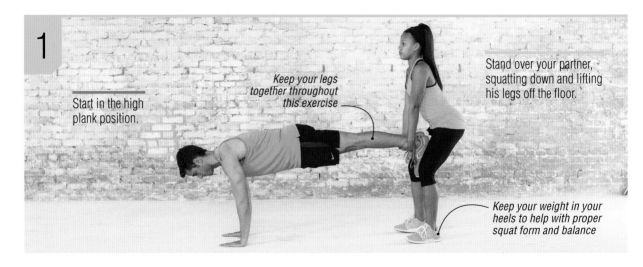

1

Start in the high plank position.

Keep your legs together throughout this exercise

Stand over your partner, squatting down and lifting his legs off the floor.

Keep your weight in your heels to help with proper squat form and balance

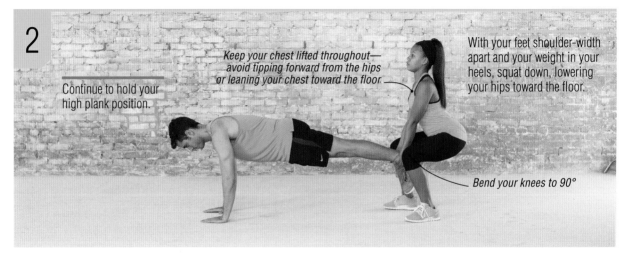

2

Continue to hold your high plank position.

Keep your chest lifted throughout—avoid tipping forward from the hips or leaning your chest toward the floor

With your feet shoulder-width apart and your weight in your heels, squat down, lowering your hips toward the floor.

Bend your knees to 90°

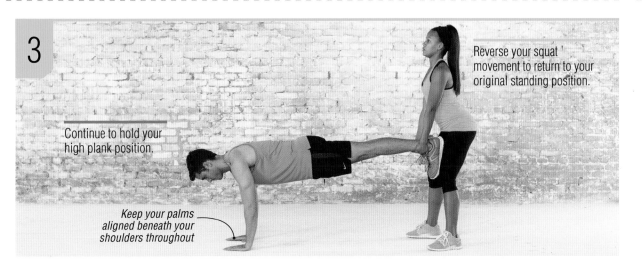

3

Reverse your squat movement to return to your original standing position.

Continue to hold your high plank position.

Keep your palms aligned beneath your shoulders throughout

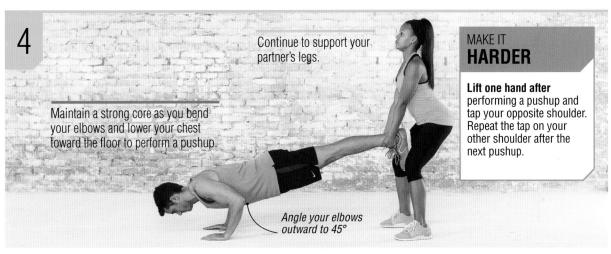

4

Continue to support your partner's legs.

Maintain a strong core as you bend your elbows and lower your chest toward the floor to perform a pushup.

Angle your elbows outward to 45°

MAKE IT
HARDER

Lift one hand after performing a pushup and tap your opposite shoulder. Repeat the tap on your other shoulder after the next pushup.

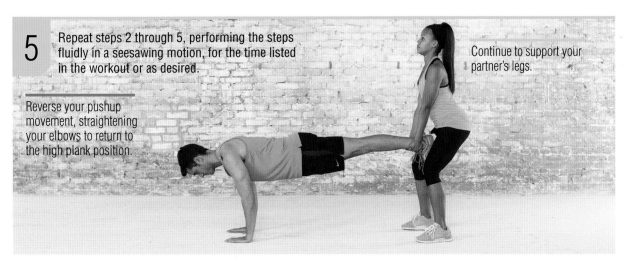

5

Repeat steps 2 through 5, performing the steps fluidly in a seesawing motion, for the time listed in the workout or as desired.

Continue to support your partner's legs.

Reverse your pushup movement, straightening your elbows to return to the high plank position.

LEVEL 2

LEG PRESS

REQUIRED EQUIPMENT   **NONE**

While performing the leg press portion of this exercise, you'll target the major muscle groups of your lower body: quads, glutes, and hamstrings. While acting as your partner's resistance, you'll use your abs, hips, and glutes to remain stable.

1

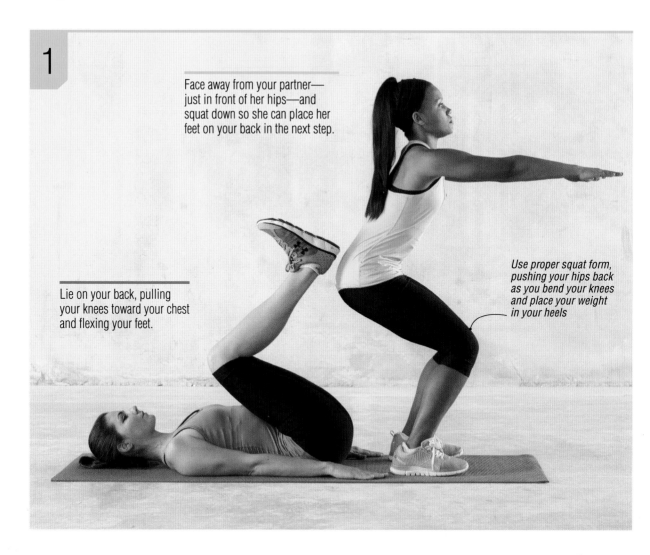

Face away from your partner—just in front of her hips—and squat down so she can place her feet on your back in the next step.

Lie on your back, pulling your knees toward your chest and flexing your feet.

Use proper squat form, pushing your hips back as you bend your knees and place your weight in your heels

2

Once your partner puts her feet on your back, cross your arms and lean into her feet as you step your feet forward until your body forms a straight line from heel to head.

Place your heels just above your partner's hips, with a foot on each side of her spine, and support your partner's weight.

VARIATION

Perform this exercise as a single-leg press by taking all the same steps but using a single leg for the leg press. Remember to switch legs to complete an equal number of reps with each leg.

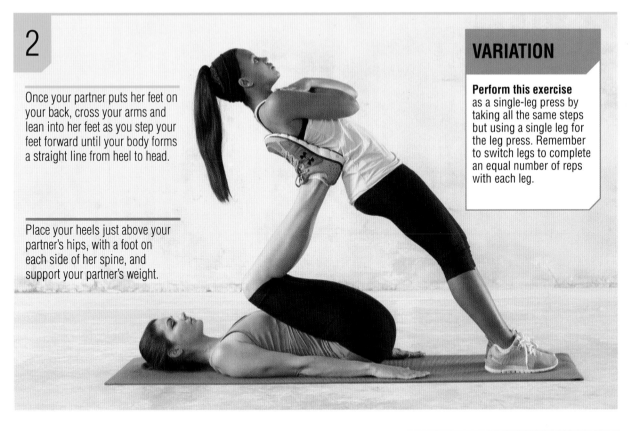

3

Tighten your abs, hips, glutes, and lower back to remain stable as your partner lifts your body.

Press your feet into your partner's back as you straighten your knees and your legs.

Keep your knees aligned with your toes—don't allow your knees to collapse inward or splay outward

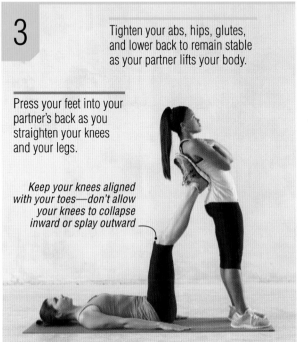

4

Repeat steps 2 through 4 for the time or reps listed in the workout or as desired.

Bend your knees, bringing them toward your chest as you work against your partner's resistance.

Maintain your position as you're lowered down.

Exhale when straightening your legs, and inhale when bringing them to your chest

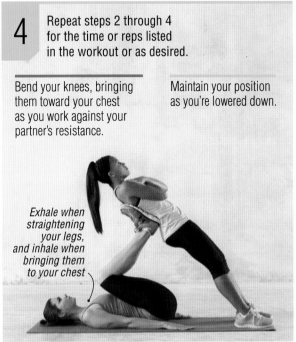

LEVEL 2

ALTERNATING GETUP

REQUIRED EQUIPMENT **NONE**

This exercise engages your glutes, core, shoulders, back, and biceps—with one partner acting as a counterbalance to the other partner's movements. You'll switch roles halfway through this exercise, transitioning fluidly between each role.

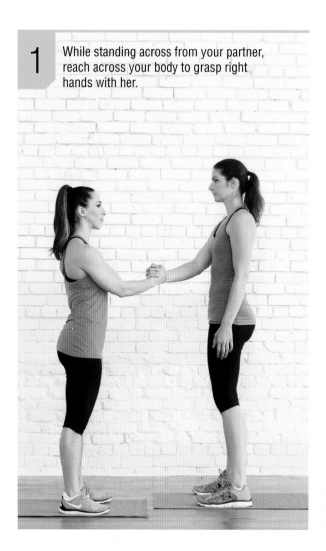

1 While standing across from your partner, reach across your body to grasp right hands with her.

2

Bend your knees, and tighten your core for support and to avoid potential injury.

Squat down, lowering your glutes toward the floor.

Continually maintain a slight bend at your elbow

3

Step toward your partner and lean forward, using your right arm and core for counterbalance support.

Use proper lunge form as you step forward, allowing your back heel to come off the floor

Roll down to a lying position.

Control your movement— don't flop backward

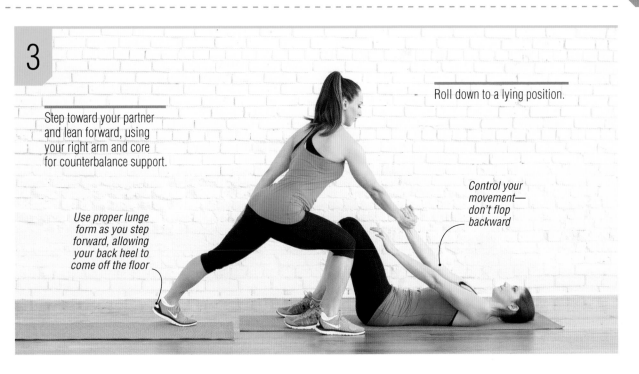

4

Roll forward while your partner pulls you to a standing position, sitting up and pushing through your heels to complete the action.

Tighten your grip to pull your partner to a standing position as you step your foot back to start.

Use your partner's arm for support as you return to standing under your own power

Your feet remain fixed to the floor throughout the downward and upward roll

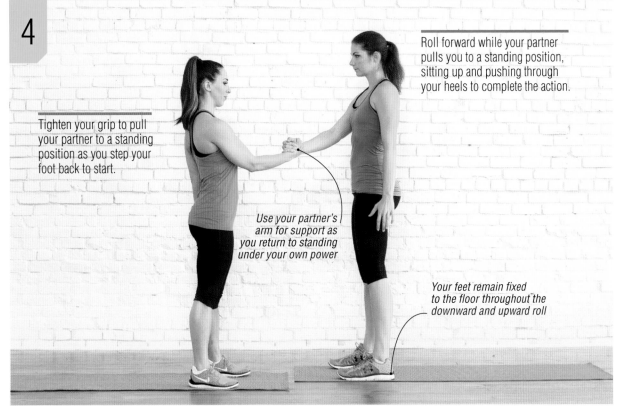

CONTINUED ••••▶

LEVEL 2

5

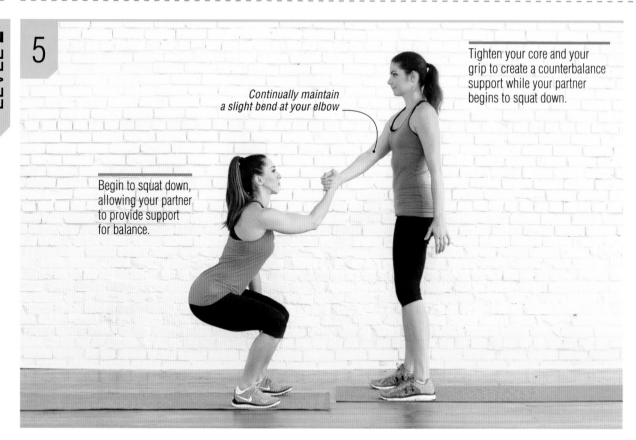

Tighten your core and your grip to create a counterbalance support while your partner begins to squat down.

Continually maintain a slight bend at your elbow

Begin to squat down, allowing your partner to provide support for balance.

6

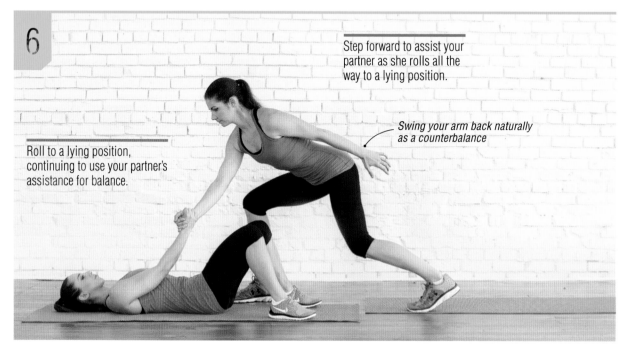

Step forward to assist your partner as she rolls all the way to a lying position.

Swing your arm back naturally as a counterbalance

Roll to a lying position, continuing to use your partner's assistance for balance.

7

Roll forward while your partner pulls you to a standing position, sitting up and pushing through your heels to regain your own balance.

Tighten your grip to pull your partner to a standing position.

MAKE IT
HARDER

Finish each getup with a squat jump. As you return to a standing position, you should jump explosively into the air.

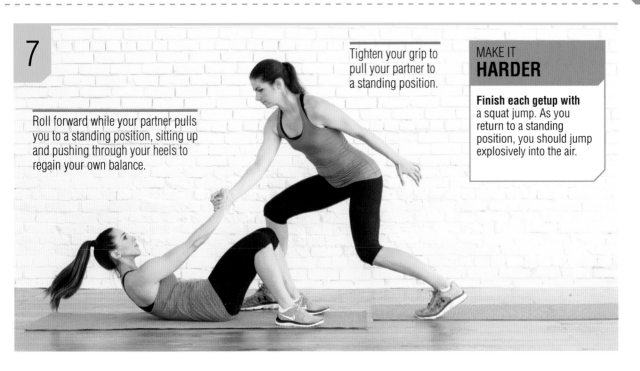

8

Maintain your grip on your partner's hand while returning to your face-to-face starting position. Repeat steps 2 through 8 for the time listed in the workout or as desired.

Keep your core tight throughout to control the movement and to help prevent a lower-back injury

Make sure your feet are roughly hip-distance apart before continuing this exercise

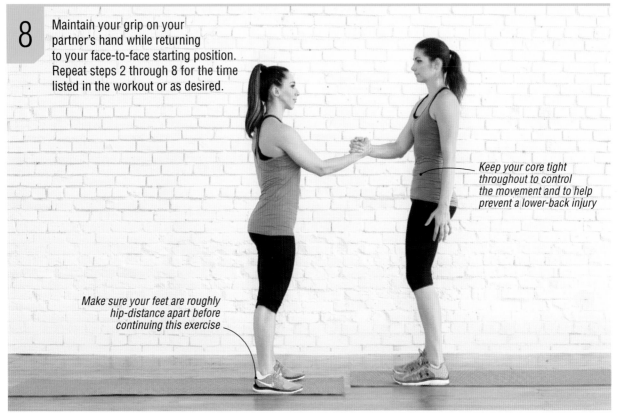

LEVEL 2

MODIFIED PULLUP

REQUIRED EQUIPMENT   **NONE**

Exercising the large muscles of the back can be tricky when you lack equipment, but all you really need is a partner. The standing partner challenges his latissimus dorsi, trapezius, and rhomboids. The partner below isometrically works her core and upper body.

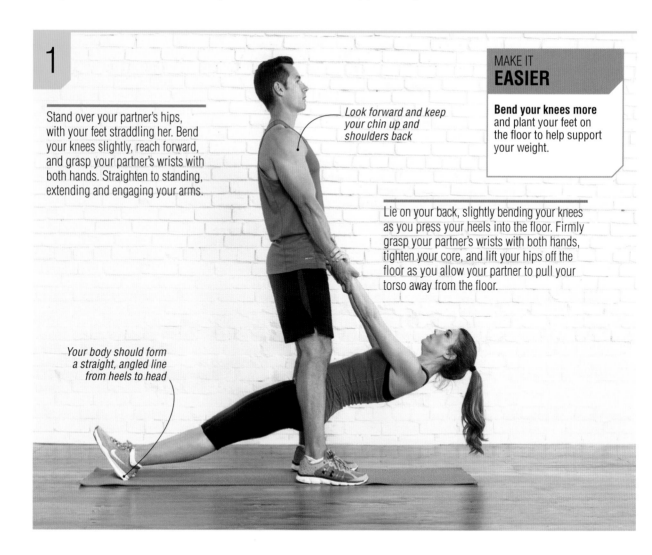

1

Stand over your partner's hips, with your feet straddling her. Bend your knees slightly, reach forward, and grasp your partner's wrists with both hands. Straighten to standing, extending and engaging your arms.

Look forward and keep your chin up and shoulders back

Your body should form a straight, angled line from heels to head

Lie on your back, slightly bending your knees as you press your heels into the floor. Firmly grasp your partner's wrists with both hands, tighten your core, and lift your hips off the floor as you allow your partner to pull your torso away from the floor.

MAKE IT EASIER

Bend your knees more and plant your feet on the floor to help support your weight.

2

Keep your knees and elbows slightly bent and muscles engaged as you lean slightly away from your partner while she performs her pullup.

Contract your abs continually, and inhale as your partner pulls up

Keep your core tight, engage your back muscles, and bend your elbows to pull yourself up toward your partner.

Keep your heels planted and your toes angled upward

Keep your elbows close to your sides

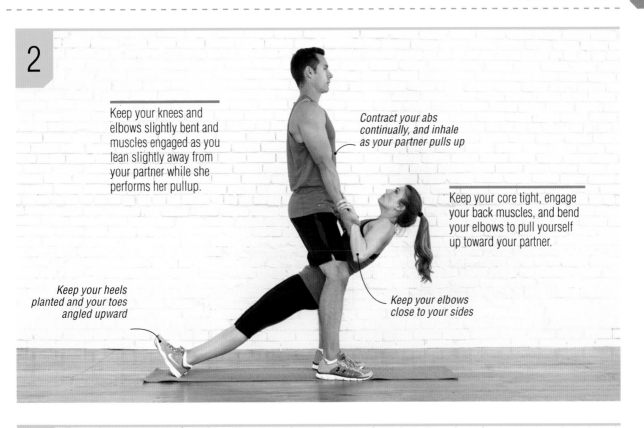

3

Repeat steps 2 and 3 for the time listed in the workout or as desired.

Keep your abs, shoulders, hips, and arms engaged to prevent hunching

Carefully reverse your movements, straightening your elbows and lowering your body toward the floor with a controlled action.

Remain upright as your partner reverses her movements and lowers herself toward the floor.

Keep your muscles engaged, and don't let gravity dictate your movements

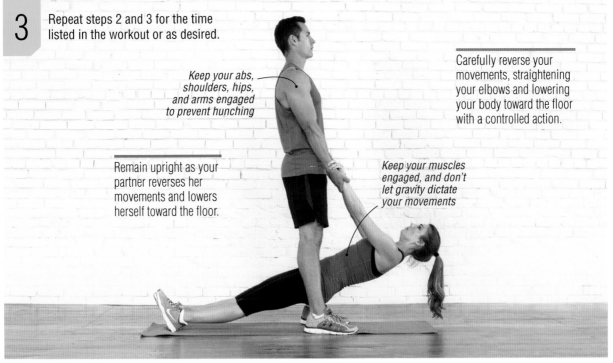

LEVEL 2

PLANK
& BENT-OVER ROW

REQUIRED EQUIPMENT   **NONE**

During this exercise, when you perform the plank, you'll challenge
your core muscles: hips, glutes, abs, lower back, chest, and shoulders.
When you execute the bent-over row, you'll work your upper back by
using your partner's body as resistance.

1

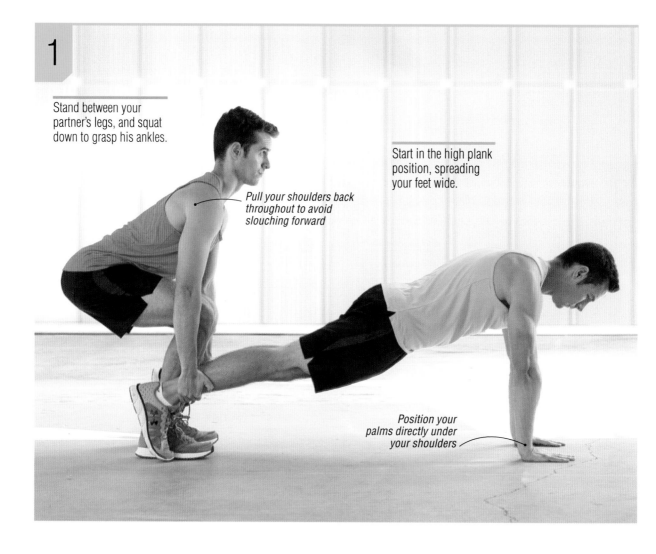

Stand between your
partner's legs, and squat
down to grasp his ankles.

Pull your shoulders back
throughout to avoid
slouching forward

Start in the high plank
position, spreading
your feet wide.

Position your
palms directly under
your shoulders

2 Return to standing as you lift your partner's legs, bending your knees slightly and hinging forward from your hips.

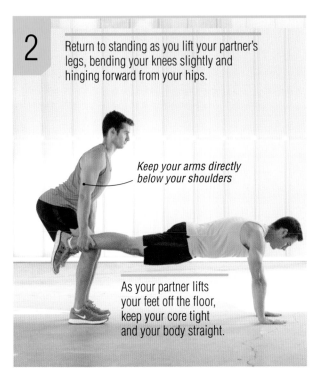

Keep your arms directly below your shoulders

As your partner lifts your feet off the floor, keep your core tight and your body straight.

3 Engage your upper back and bend your elbows, pulling them up to your sides and lifting your partner's legs to hip height.

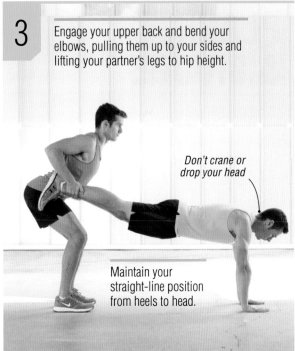

Don't crane or drop your head

Maintain your straight-line position from heels to head.

4 Repeat steps 3 and 4 for the time listed in the workout or as desired.

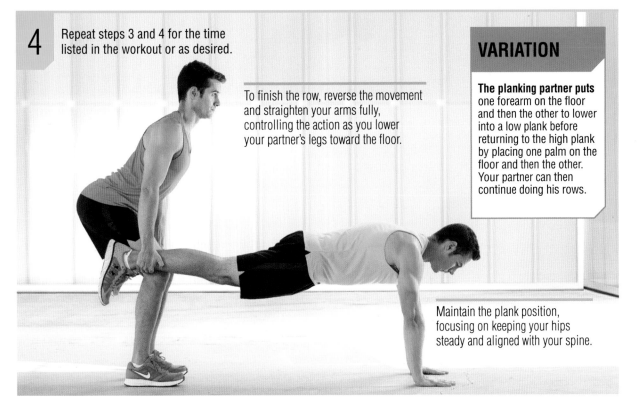

To finish the row, reverse the movement and straighten your arms fully, controlling the action as you lower your partner's legs toward the floor.

VARIATION

The planking partner puts one forearm on the floor and then the other to lower into a low plank before returning to the high plank by placing one palm on the floor and then the other. Your partner can then continue doing his rows.

Maintain the plank position, focusing on keeping your hips steady and aligned with your spine.

PLANK & BRIDGE

REQUIRED EQUIPMENT **NONE**

During this paired exercise, both partners work their core muscles—but in slightly different ways. While in the plank, you'll target the front of your body, and when you perform the bridge, you'll work the muscles on the back of your body.

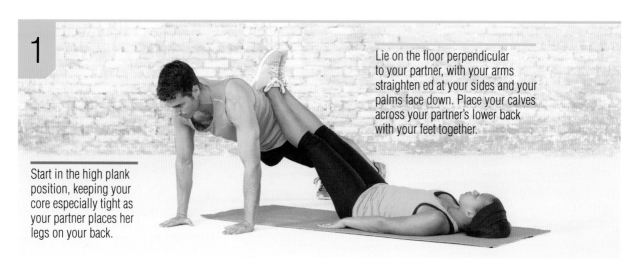

1

Lie on the floor perpendicular to your partner, with your arms straighten ed at your sides and your palms face down. Place your calves across your partner's lower back with your feet together.

Start in the high plank position, keeping your core especially tight as your partner places her legs on your back.

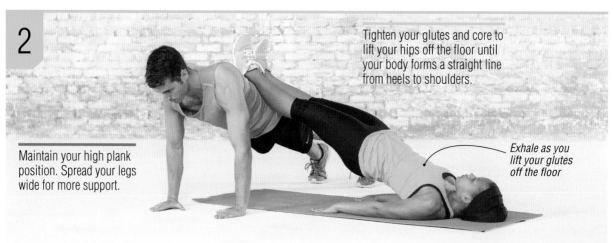

2

Tighten your glutes and core to lift your hips off the floor until your body forms a straight line from heels to shoulders.

Maintain your high plank position. Spread your legs wide for more support.

Exhale as you lift your glutes off the floor

3

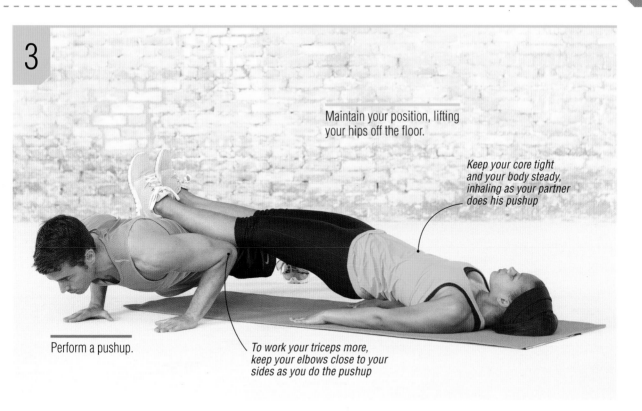

Maintain your position, lifting your hips off the floor.

Keep your core tight and your body steady, inhaling as your partner does his pushup

Perform a pushup.

To work your triceps more, keep your elbows close to your sides as you do the pushup

4

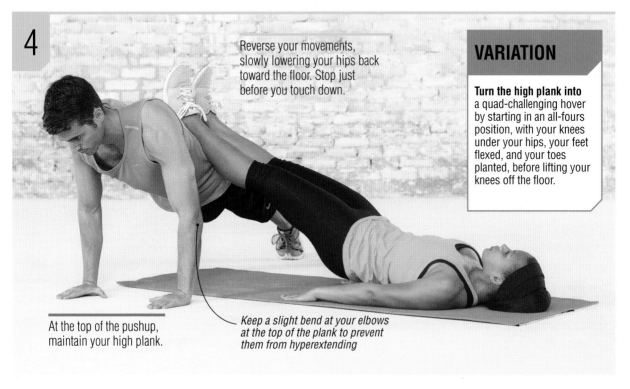

Reverse your movements, slowly lowering your hips back toward the floor. Stop just before you touch down.

VARIATION

Turn the high plank into a quad-challenging hover by starting in an all-fours position, with your knees under your hips, your feet flexed, and your toes planted, before lifting your knees off the floor.

At the top of the pushup, maintain your high plank.

Keep a slight bend at your elbows at the top of the plank to prevent them from hyperextending

LEVEL 2

BRIDGE HOLD & DIP

REQUIRED EQUIPMENT **NONE**

Both partners will work different muscle groups. The isometric (static) bridge targets the core, glutes, and hamstrings, and the triceps dip focuses on the backs of the arms and shoulders while also engaging the abs, hips, glutes, and quads to help control the movement.

1

Facing away from your partner, squat down to place one hand on each of your partner's knees, fully straightening your arms. Step your legs out until they're also straightened and you're in a suspended sitting position.

MAKE IT EASIER

While in the suspended sitting position, bend your knees and plant your feet flat to help support your weight rather than straighten them.

Get into bridge position by lying on your back, with your knees bent and your feet planted hip-distance apart. Engage your core and glutes to push your hips up until your body forms a straight line from your knees to your shoulders.

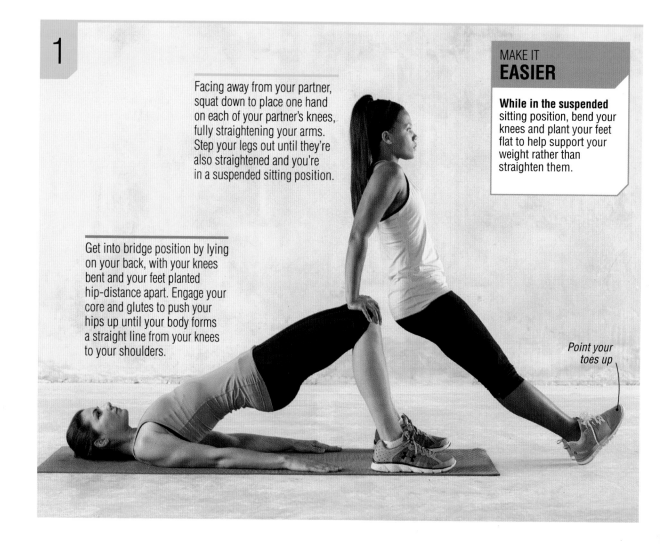

Point your toes up

2

Stop when your elbows are at 90°

Perform a dip by bending your elbows, and at a steady pace, lower your hips toward the floor by contracting your triceps, core, and shoulders.

Maintain your bridge position, pushing your hips as high up as you can.

Drop your hips straight down toward the floor

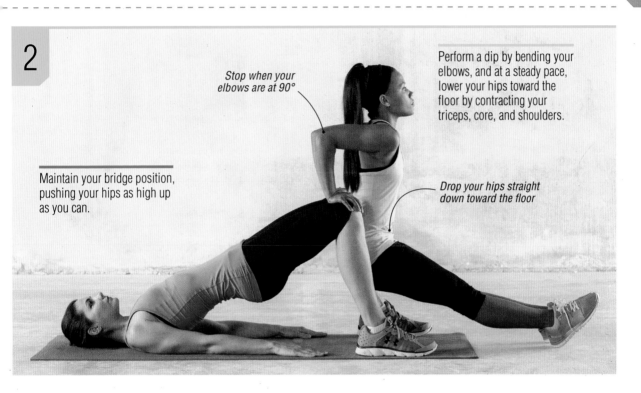

3

Repeat steps 2 and 3 for the time listed in the workout or as desired.

Keep your shoulders engaged and pulled back so your shoulders don't shrug up toward your ears

Press your palms against your partner's knees to reverse your movements, and straighten your elbows to return to your starting position.

Continue to maintain your bridge position.

Press your arms and hands into the floor for added support

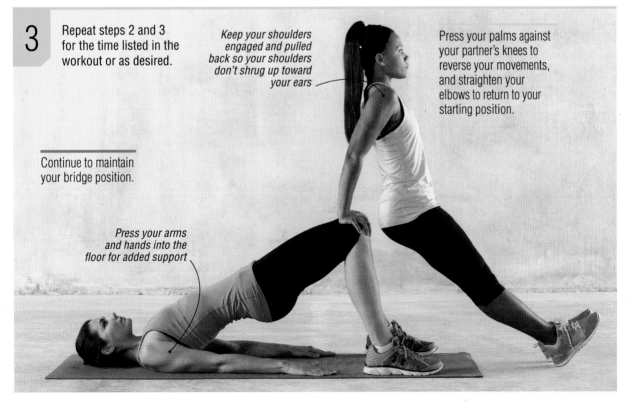

V-SIT ADDUCTOR & ABDUCTOR

REQUIRED EQUIPMENT **NONE**

The leg adductors and abductors are the muscles that help move your legs back and forth sideways. For this exercise, both partners will challenge their inner and outer thigh muscles by working together to provide resistance for each other.

1 Sit facing each other, with one partner's legs just outside the other partner's legs. Lean back, placing your palms on the floor behind you for support, bending your elbows, and keeping your torso engaged and straight.

MAKE IT EASIER

If maintaining a V is too hard, plant one foot on the floor, keeping your knee bent, and do this exercise one leg at a time.

Lift your legs up so they form a V with your body, slightly spreading them so your inner ankles touch your partner's outer ankles.

Keep your ankles together so your partner's inner ankles touch your outer ankles as you lift your legs up into a V shape.

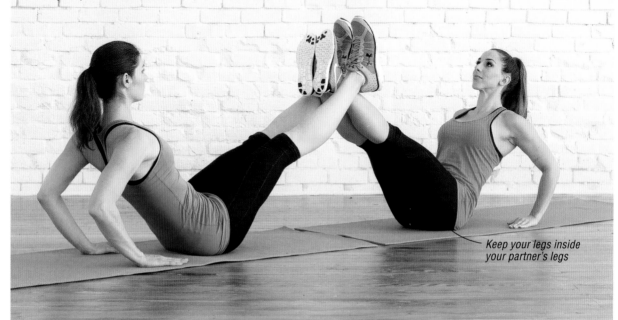

Keep your legs inside your partner's legs

2

Engage your inner thighs and resist your partner as she tries to abduct (spread) her legs wide. Resist—but still allow the movement.

Press your legs outward against your partner's resistance as you try to spread your legs as wide as possible.

Keep your shoulders back to prevent slouching

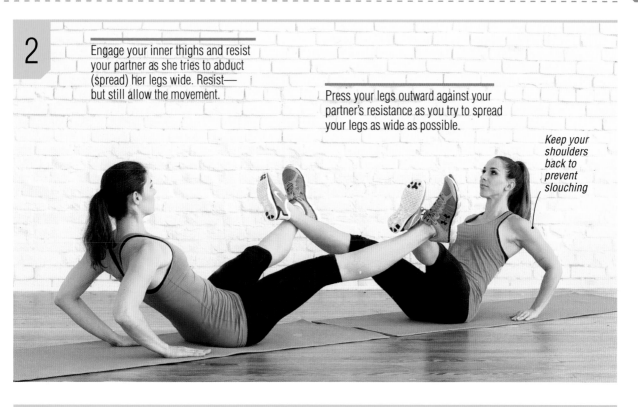

3

Press inward with both legs, trying to pull your thighs together against your partner's resistance.

Engage your outer thighs and glutes to provide resistance for your partner, working to slow the movement as she pulls her thighs together.

Keep your abs and lower back contracted throughout

Your upper thighs will feel the burn

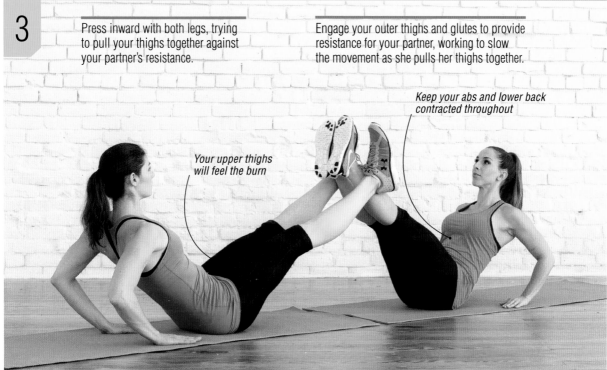

ASSISTED PISTOL SQUAT

REQUIRED EQUIPMENT **NONE**

A pistol squat is an advanced move that targets all the muscles of your lower body unilaterally—one side at a time. When performing the squat with a partner, it's still an advanced move, but you can use your partner's support to help you master proper form.

1 Stand facing your partner, and reach your right hand across your body to grasp his forearm just above the wrist. Straighten your left leg forward, with your knee straight.

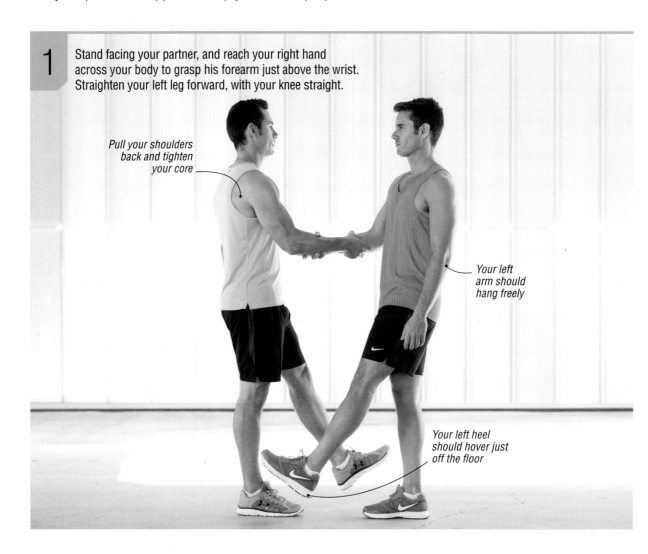

Pull your shoulders back and tighten your core

Your left arm should hang freely

Your left heel should hover just off the floor

2

Working in tandem, push your hips back, bend your supporting knee, and squat down, aiming to touch the hamstrings of your supporting leg to your calf, with your glutes just off the floor.

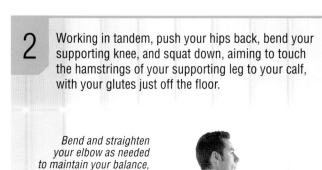

Bend and straighten your elbow as needed to maintain your balance, but use your partner for support

Keep your nonsupporting leg straight throughout

Keep your weight in your heel to maintain your balance and support proper form

MAKE IT
HARDER

At the bottom of your first squat, lean forward and grasp the toes of your straightened leg, extending it completely so it's parallel to the floor. Perform subsequent pistol squats while holding your toes.

3

Push through your supporting heel, leaning forward slightly as you return to standing. Repeat steps 2 and 3 for the time listed in the workout or as desired.

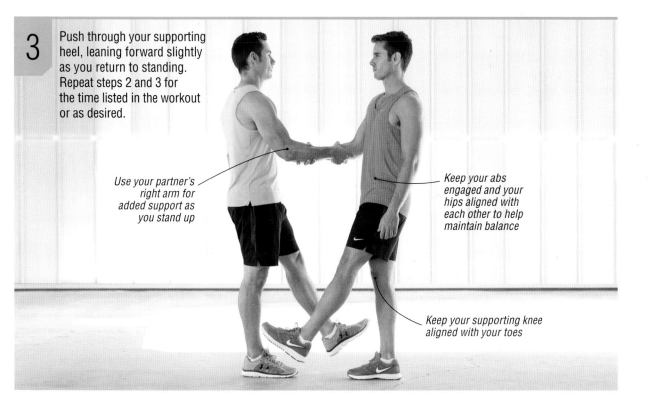

Use your partner's right arm for added support as you stand up

Keep your abs engaged and your hips aligned with each other to help maintain balance

Keep your supporting knee aligned with your toes

WALL SQUAT
& BULGARIAN SPLIT SQUAT

REQUIRED EQUIPMENT   **NONE**

While the isometric wall squat won't be easy, it's actually the easier element of this lower-body move. While both partners target their glutes, hamstrings, quads, and calves, the partner doing the Bulgarian split squat has the added challenge of a plyometric jumping exercise.

1 Stand facing away from your partner. Lift your right foot and bend your right knee, placing your lifted ankle across your partner's right thigh.

Lean against a wall with your feet hip-distance apart. Step your feet forward slightly before sliding your hips down to form 90° angles at your hips and knees.

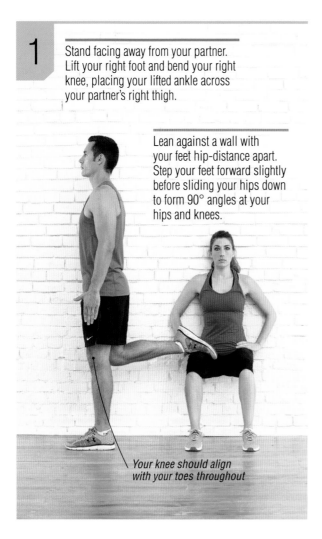

Your knee should align with your toes throughout

2 Bend your supporting knee, lowering yourself into a single-leg squat. Keeping your torso straight and core engaged, lean forward to reach your hands toward the floor on either side of your supporting leg.

Maintain your wall squat position, keeping your hips and back flush with the wall.

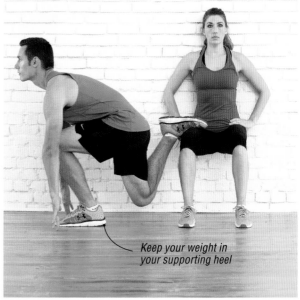

Keep your weight in your supporting heel

3 With explosive power, forcefully push through your supporting foot from heel to toe, springing into the air as you straighten your supporting leg.

MAKE IT
EASIER

The jumping partner doesn't need to jump all the way into the air—simply rising up on your toes can help improve power.

Maintain your wall squat position, keeping your hips and torso pressing into the wall.

Push your arms backward to help your upward propulsion

Only jump as high as you comfortably can

The leg supporting your partner might move as he jumps, but keep your hips and torso steady

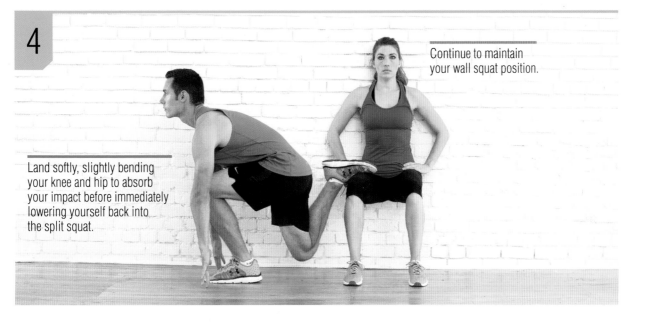

4

Continue to maintain your wall squat position.

Land softly, slightly bending your knee and hip to absorb your impact before immediately lowering yourself back into the split squat.

LEVEL 3

KNEELING HAMSTRING CURLS

REQUIRED EQUIPMENT **NONE**

This exercise might look easy, but it's surprisingly hard. Make sure you're properly warmed up before you dive into this move. In addition to working his. hamstrings, the active partner also challenges his core, chest, and triceps.

1

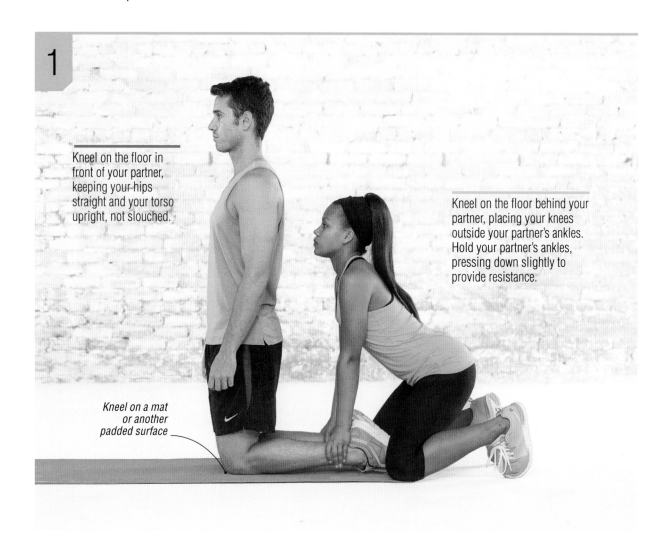

Kneel on the floor in front of your partner, keeping your hips straight and your torso upright, not slouched.

Kneel on the floor behind your partner, placing your knees outside your partner's ankles. Hold your partner's ankles, pressing down slightly to provide resistance.

Kneel on a mat or another padded surface

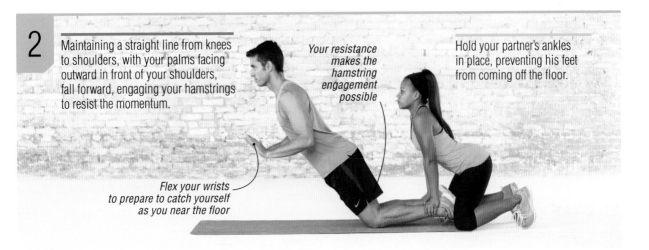

2 Maintaining a straight line from knees to shoulders, with your palms facing outward in front of your shoulders, fall forward, engaging your hamstrings to resist the momentum.

Your resistance makes the hamstring engagement possible

Hold your partner's ankles in place, preventing his feet from coming off the floor.

Flex your wrists to prepare to catch yourself as you near the floor

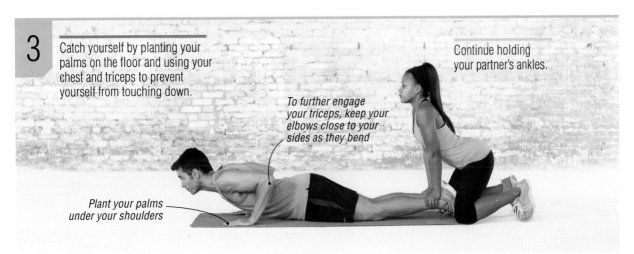

3 Catch yourself by planting your palms on the floor and using your chest and triceps to prevent yourself from touching down.

To further engage your triceps, keep your elbows close to your sides as they bend

Continue holding your partner's ankles.

Plant your palms under your shoulders

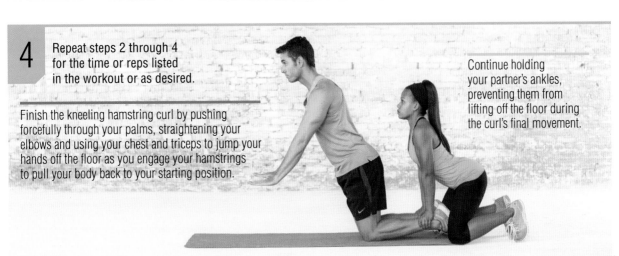

4 Repeat steps 2 through 4 for the time or reps listed in the workout or as desired.

Finish the kneeling hamstring curl by pushing forcefully through your palms, straightening your elbows and using your chest and triceps to jump your hands off the floor as you engage your hamstrings to pull your body back to your starting position.

Continue holding your partner's ankles, preventing them from lifting off the floor during the curl's final movement.

TWISTING SQUAT & BOSU PUSHUP

REQUIRED EQUIPMENT **MEDICINE BALL • BOSU BALL**

This multifaceted exercise works just about everything from head to toe. One partner challenges the lower body and core with a twisting wall squat, while the other works on upper-body strength and balance with a BOSU pushup. Pairing them, they offer double the effects.

1

Position yourself in the high plank, placing your shins across your partner's thighs as you place your hands on the BOSU ball.

Place the BOSU on the floor, dome side down

Lean against a wall, holding the medicine ball in front of your chest. Slide your hips down the wall until your knees and hips are at 90°.

Keep your feet shoulder-width apart

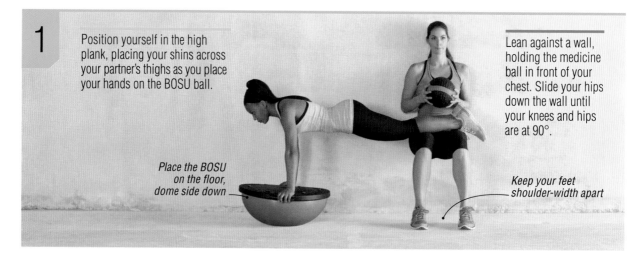

2

Keep your core tight, bend your elbows, and engage your chest and triceps, lowering your chest toward the BOSU.

Bend your right elbow and keep it close to your side

Maintaining your squat and keeping your hips steady, twist your torso to the right, tapping the ball on the wall.

Lower yourself until you almost touch the BOSU

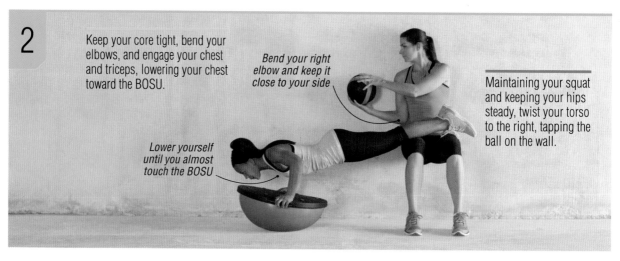

3

VARIATION

The partner working with the BOSU can put one knee forward and to the outside of the same-side elbow while lowering her chest toward the BOSU. Alternate sides with each pushup.

Keeping your hips fixed to the wall, twist your torso back toward center, but this time, turn all the way across to tap the ball on the wall on your left side.

Press through your palms, straightening your elbows as you push yourself back to your starting position.

Perform the oblique twist at your own speed— it doesn't need to be done in sync with your partner

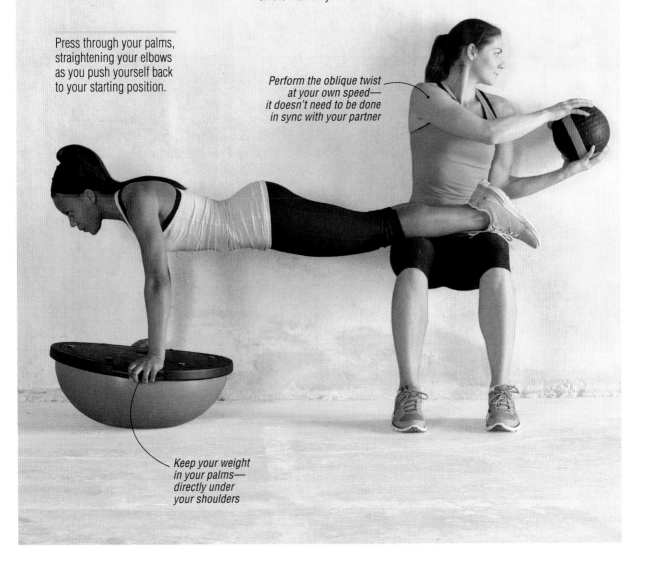

Keep your weight in your palms— directly under your shoulders

SITUP TO SQUARE PIKE

REQUIRED EQUIPMENT **NONE**

When you're looking for a core challenge, you can't get much more demanding than this exercise. Both partners will work their abs while also benefitting from an added dose of shoulder and chest work. Go slow—and take the time to master proper form.

1

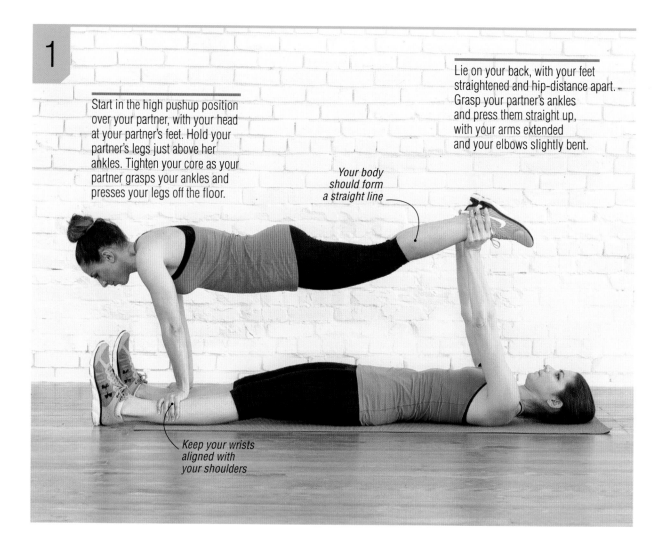

Start in the high pushup position over your partner, with your head at your partner's feet. Hold your partner's legs just above her ankles. Tighten your core as your partner grasps your ankles and presses your legs off the floor.

Lie on your back, with your feet straightened and hip-distance apart. Grasp your partner's ankles and press them straight up, with your arms extended and your elbows slightly bent.

Your body should form a straight line

Keep your wrists aligned with your shoulders

2

Engage your core, lifting your hips as you move into a piked handstand, with your body forming an upside-down L.

At the top of this exercise, your hips should be bent at 90°

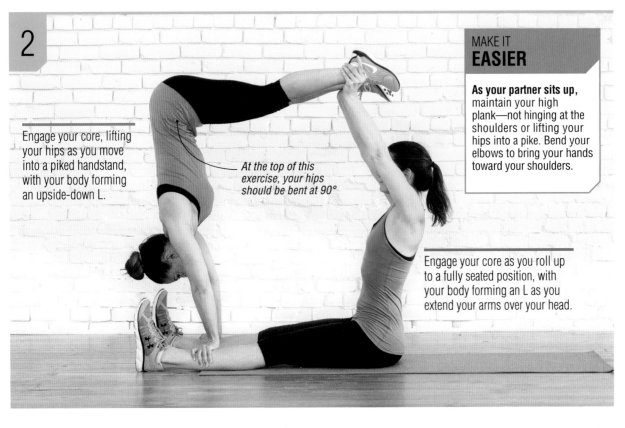

MAKE IT
EASIER

As your partner sits up, maintain your high plank—not hinging at the shoulders or lifting your hips into a pike. Bend your elbows to bring your hands toward your shoulders.

Engage your core as you roll up to a fully seated position, with your body forming an L as you extend your arms over your head.

3

As your partner rolls down to the floor, carefully reverse your movements, lowering your hips and pulling your head forward to return to your starting position.

Keeping your arms straight to help support your partner, roll your body back down to return to your starting position.

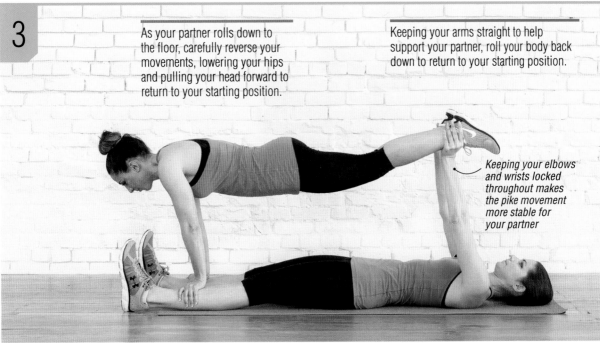

Keeping your elbows and wrists locked throughout makes the pike movement more stable for your partner

LEVEL 3

HANDSTAND SHOULDER PRESS

REQUIRED EQUIPMENT **NONE**

This exercise requires strength, courage—and trust. You need strength in your shoulders, the courage to flip upside down, and the trust that your partner won't allow you to fall. While you'll definitely work your shoulders, you should also feel your abs, back, and hips help stabilize your body.

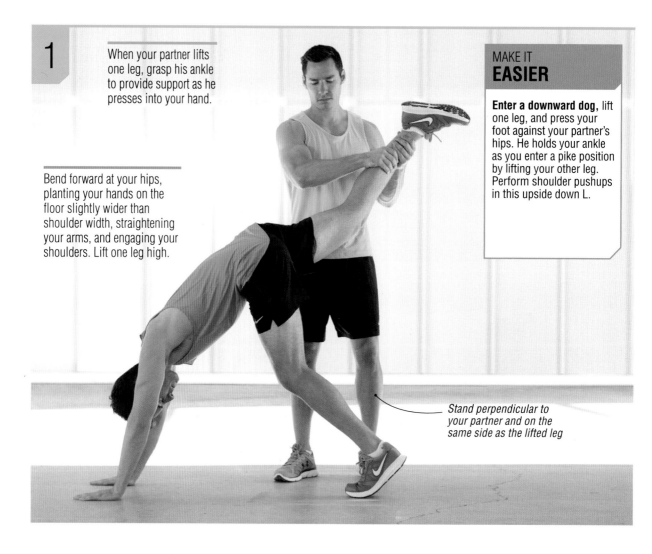

1

When your partner lifts one leg, grasp his ankle to provide support as he presses into your hand.

Bend forward at your hips, planting your hands on the floor slightly wider than shoulder width, straightening your arms, and engaging your shoulders. Lift one leg high.

MAKE IT
EASIER

Enter a downward dog, lift one leg, and press your foot against your partner's hips. He holds your ankle as you enter a pike position by lifting your other leg. Perform shoulder pushups in this upside down L.

Stand perpendicular to your partner and on the same side as the lifted leg

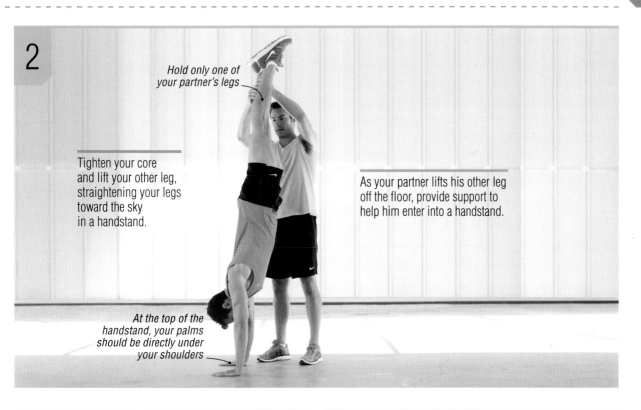

2

Hold only one of your partner's legs

Tighten your core and lift your other leg, straightening your legs toward the sky in a handstand.

As your partner lifts his other leg off the floor, provide support to help him enter into a handstand.

At the top of the handstand, your palms should be directly under your shoulders

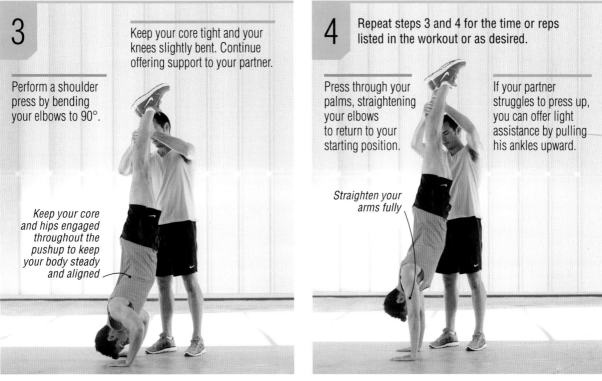

3

Keep your core tight and your knees slightly bent. Continue offering support to your partner.

Perform a shoulder press by bending your elbows to 90°.

Keep your core and hips engaged throughout the pushup to keep your body steady and aligned

4

Repeat steps 3 and 4 for the time or reps listed in the workout or as desired.

Press through your palms, straightening your elbows to return to your starting position.

If your partner struggles to press up, you can offer light assistance by pulling his ankles upward.

Straighten your arms fully

LEVEL 3

ELEVATED PUSHUP & CHEST PRESS

REQUIRED EQUIPMENT **NONE**

This exercise offers double the chest workout and double the fun, with each partner strengthening the pectoral muscles in different ways. While you target your chest, core, and triceps, you'll also share some laughs while trying to stay in position for resistance and support.

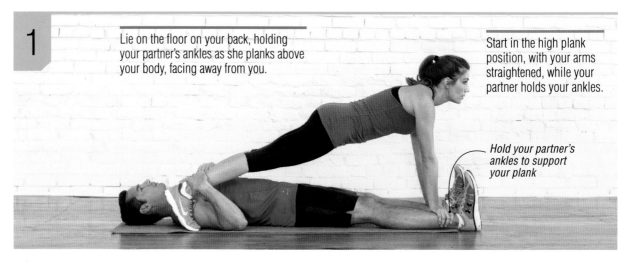

1

Lie on the floor on your back, holding your partner's ankles as she planks above your body, facing away from you.

Start in the high plank position, with your arms straightened, while your partner holds your ankles.

Hold your partner's ankles to support your plank

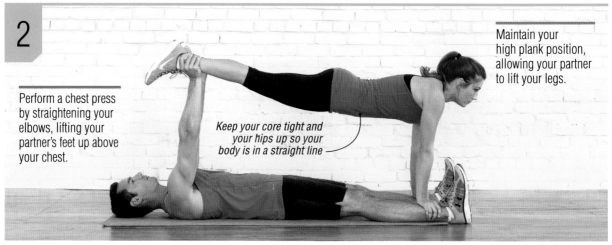

2

Maintain your high plank position, allowing your partner to lift your legs.

Perform a chest press by straightening your elbows, lifting your partner's feet up above your chest.

Keep your core tight and your hips up so your body is in a straight line

3

Lower your partner's feet toward your chest, stopping just before your elbows touch the floor.

Bend your elbows to 90° to lower into the bottom part of a pushup while allowing your partner to lower your legs at the same time.

Stop just before your chest touches your partner's legs

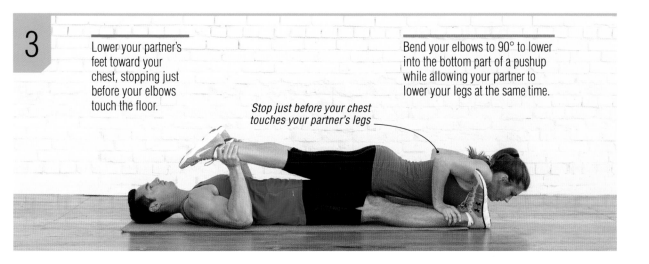

4

Repeat steps 3 and 4 for the time listed in the workout or as desired.

Straighten your elbows, raising your chest back off the floor into the top position of a pushup.

Lift your partner's legs back above your chest, straightening your elbows.

MAKE IT EASIER

Eliminate the pushup and simply hold the high plank while your partner performs the chest press with your legs.

Keep your abs engaged, pressing your lower back into the floor

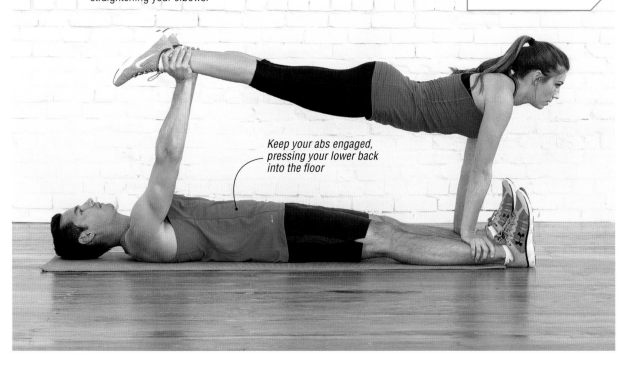

LEVEL 3

ASSISTED PLYOMETRIC BULGARIAN SPLIT SQUAT

REQUIRED EQUIPMENT   **NONE**

This exercise will challenge your lower-body power and strength while boosting your heart rate. And if that's not enough, this exercise also requires balance and core strength as you jump from and land on a single leg.

1 Stand facing the same direction as your partner, with one of you in front of the other.

Shift your weight to one side, lifting your opposite foot, bending your knee, and placing your foot in your partner's cupped hands.

Interlace your fingers, straighten your arms between your legs, and squat down slightly, using your cupped hands to support your partner's foot.

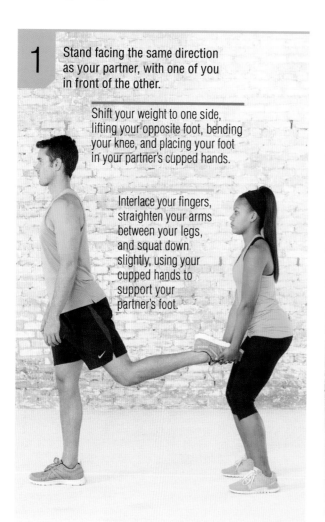

2 Tighten your core, bend both knees, and reach your hands toward the floor on either side of your front foot as you lean forward slightly. Keep your weight in the heel of your front foot.

Maintain your support position.

Keep your core tight

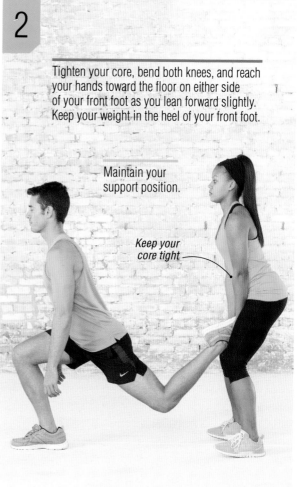

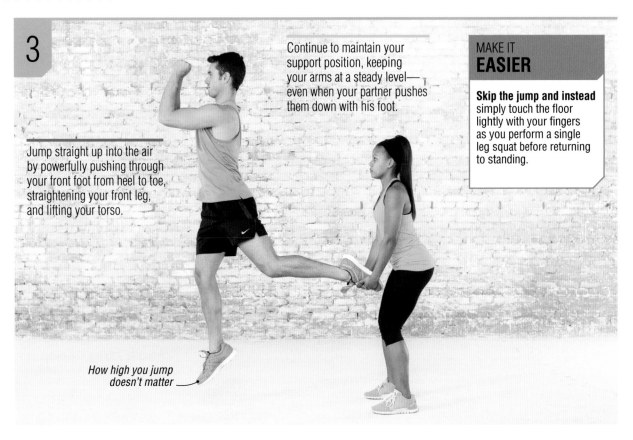

3

Jump straight up into the air by powerfully pushing through your front foot from heel to toe, straightening your front leg, and lifting your torso.

Continue to maintain your support position, keeping your arms at a steady level—even when your partner pushes them down with his foot.

How high you jump doesn't matter

MAKE IT
EASIER

Skip the jump and instead simply touch the floor lightly with your fingers as you perform a single leg squat before returning to standing.

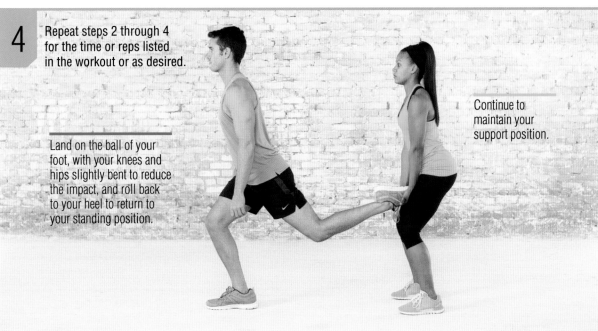

4

Repeat steps 2 through 4 for the time or reps listed in the workout or as desired.

Land on the ball of your foot, with your knees and hips slightly bent to reduce the impact, and roll back to your heel to return to your standing position.

Continue to maintain your support position.

LEVEL 3

DOUBLE BRIDGE

REQUIRED EQUIPMENT **NONE**

This exercise will challenge your glutes and hamstrings while also requiring balance and core strength to master the movements. Communicate with your partner to stay in sync—and to maximize results while minimizing any potential for injury.

1 Sit facing each other before lying on your backs, with your knees bent and your feet flat on the floor. Lift your feet off the floor and bend your knees to 90°, touching the soles of your feet to the soles of your partner's feet.

MAKE IT HARDER

Isolate one leg at a time by crossing one ankle over the opposite knee before pressing your supporting foot into your partner's foot (right foot to right foot or left foot to left foot). Once situated, perform the bridge using one leg.

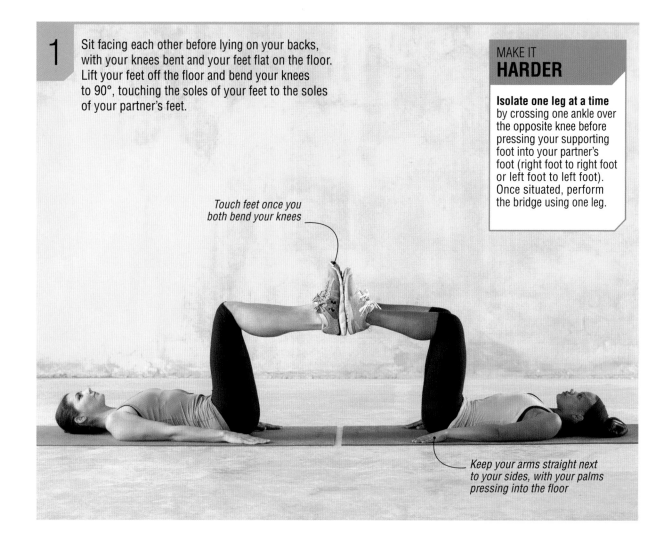

Touch feet once you both bend your knees

Keep your arms straight next to your sides, with your palms pressing into the floor

2 Press into each other's feet for support, and engage your cores as you lift your hips, pushing them up until your bodies form a straight line from shoulders to knees.

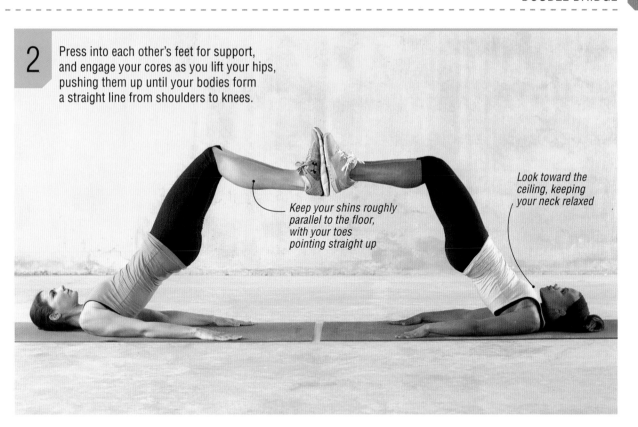

Keep your shins roughly parallel to the floor, with your toes pointing straight up

Look toward the ceiling, keeping your neck relaxed

3 Lower your hips back toward the floor, stopping just before you touch down. Repeat steps 2 and 3 for the time listed in the workout or as desired.

Keep a lot of pressure on your feet and shoulders for balance and support

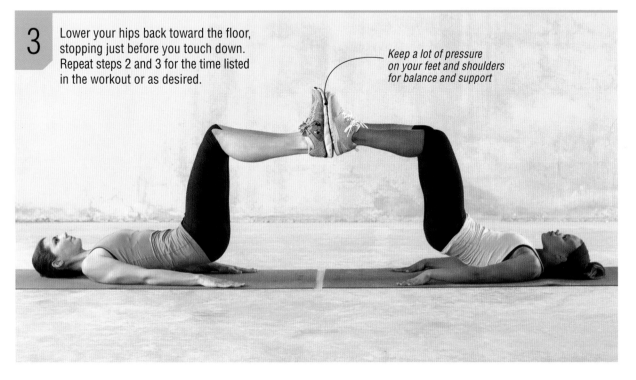

WEIGHTED PLANK & LATERAL HOPS

REQUIRED EQUIPMENT **NONE**

This advanced conditioning exercise requires serious lower-body power and core strength. You'll actually use your partner's body like a hurdle as you hop back and forth across it. Plus, by placing your weight across your partner's shoulders, you'll also make your partner's plank tougher.

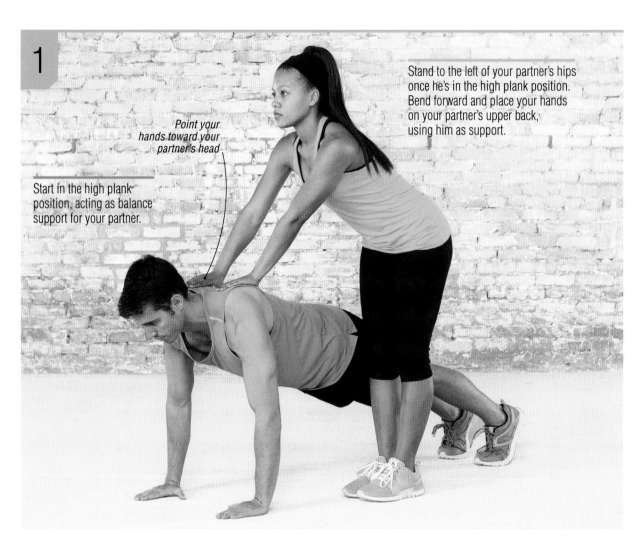

1

Point your hands toward your partner's head

Start in the high plank position, acting as balance support for your partner.

Stand to the left of your partner's hips once he's in the high plank position. Bend forward and place your hands on your partner's upper back, using him as support.

2 Engage your core and explosively jump sideways over your partner.

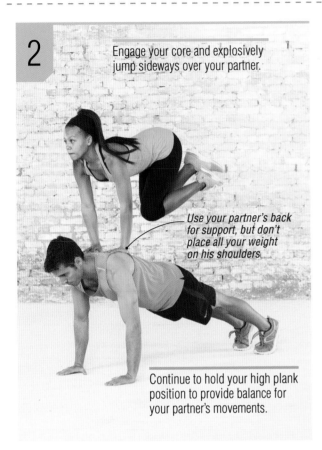

Use your partner's back for support, but don't place all your weight on his shoulders

Continue to hold your high plank position to provide balance for your partner's movements.

3 Land on your feet to your partner's right side, slightly bending your knees to absorb the impact as you land.

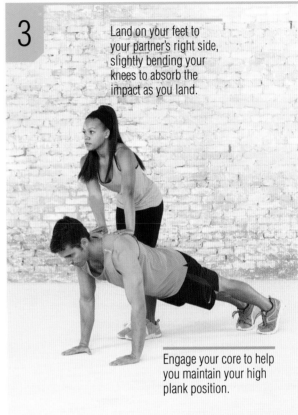

Engage your core to help you maintain your high plank position.

4 Repeat steps 2 through 4 for the time listed in the workout or as desired.

Immediately hop into the air, propelling yourself up and over to the left. Land on your feet slightly to the left of your partner.

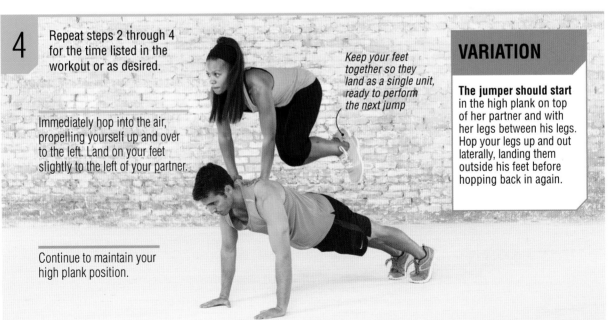

Keep your feet together so they land as a single unit, ready to perform the next jump

Continue to maintain your high plank position.

VARIATION

The jumper should start in the high plank on top of her partner and with her legs between his legs. Hop your legs up and out laterally, landing them outside his feet before hopping back in again.

LEVEL 3

LINKED-LEG PUSHUPS

REQUIRED EQUIPMENT **NONE**

Pushups are an excellent way to work your upper body and core, but your legs usually play a role in supporting your weight. With this modified exercise, you'll rely on your chest, shoulder, triceps, and core strength—with the added challenge of supporting your partner's weight.

1 Start in the high plank position, facing away from each other, with one partner's legs together and the other partner's legs positioned outside his partner's legs.

MAKE IT **EASIER**

One partner maintains the high plank, with feet on his partner's shoulders to add weight, while the other partner keeps his feet on the floor while performing pushups.

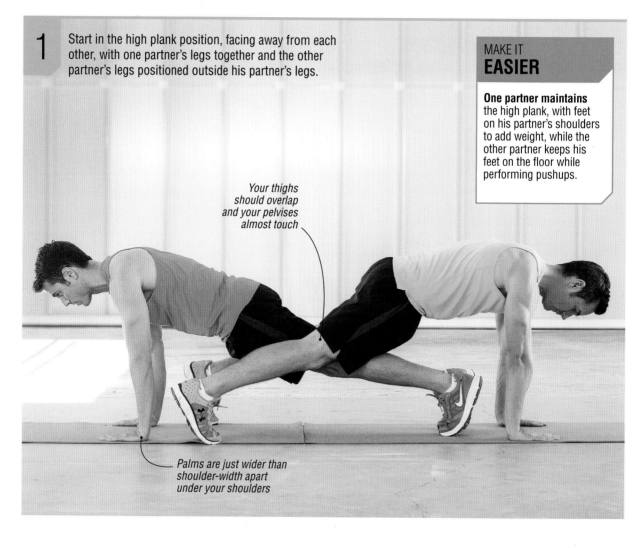

Your thighs should overlap and your pelvises almost touch

Palms are just wider than shoulder-width apart under your shoulders

2 Tighten your cores, and place your feet—one at a time— on your partner's shoulder blades, positioning yourselves into shoulder pushup position.

Avoid craning your neck or arching your back

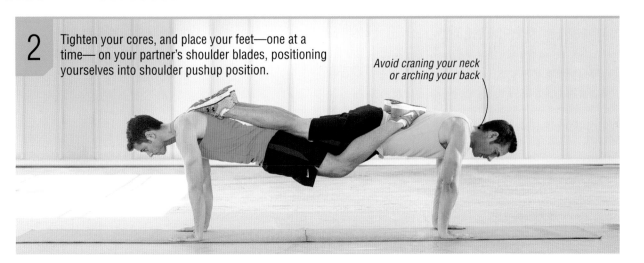

3 As a unit, bend your elbows and lower your chests toward the floor.

Stop when your elbows are at 90°

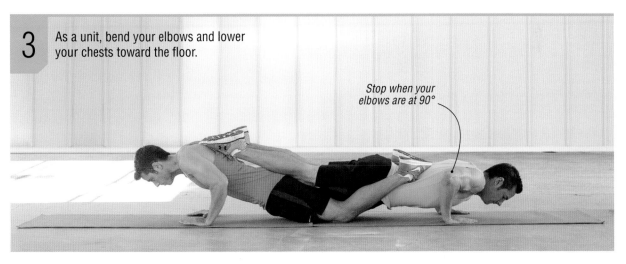

4 As a unit, straighten your arms to return to your high plank positions. Repeat steps 3 and 4 for the time listed in the workout or as desired.

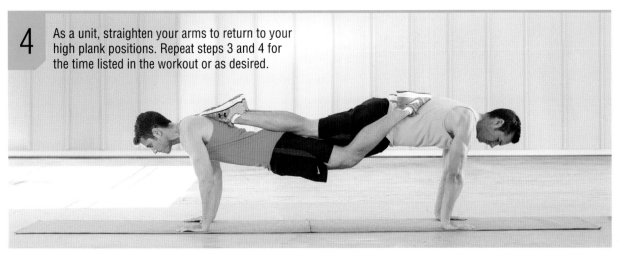

FIREMAN'S CARRY

REQUIRED EQUIPMENT **NONE**

You haven't experienced a truly challenging exercise until you've tried walking any distance with someone balanced across your shoulders. When you're the carrier, this exercise will make your whole body burn as you develop cardiovascular and muscular endurance.

1

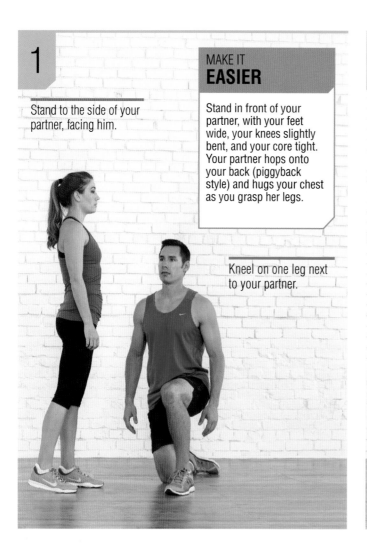

Stand to the side of your partner, facing him.

Kneel on one leg next to your partner.

MAKE IT EASIER

Stand in front of your partner, with your feet wide, your knees slightly bent, and your core tight. Your partner hops onto your back (piggyback style) and hugs your chest as you grasp her legs.

2

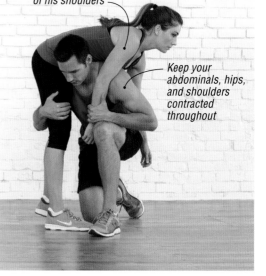

Allow your partner to grab you around your legs and arms, lifting you as he stands up.

Grasp around your partner's legs and arms to secure her across your shoulders before you powerfully push through your front heel to stand up.

Put one arm across your partner's back and the other in front of his shoulders

Keep your abdominals, hips, and shoulders contracted throughout

3 Stand up and walk forward as fast as you comfortably can, keeping your partner steady across your shoulders, until you meet your time, steps, or distance goal.

Keep your body as steady as possible to help your partner with his balance— and to help prevent him from dropping you.

4 Prepare to stand as your partner puts you back on the floor.

Once you meet your goal, carefully lunge forward to put your partner on the floor.

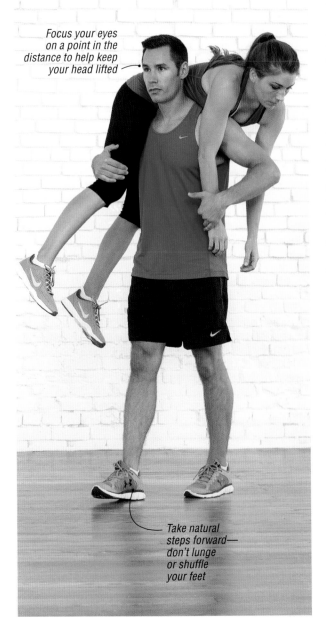

Focus your eyes on a point in the distance to help keep your head lifted

Take natural steps forward— don't lunge or shuffle your feet

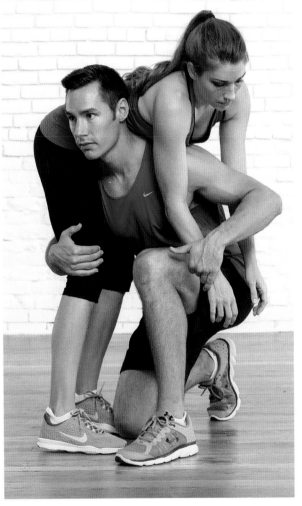

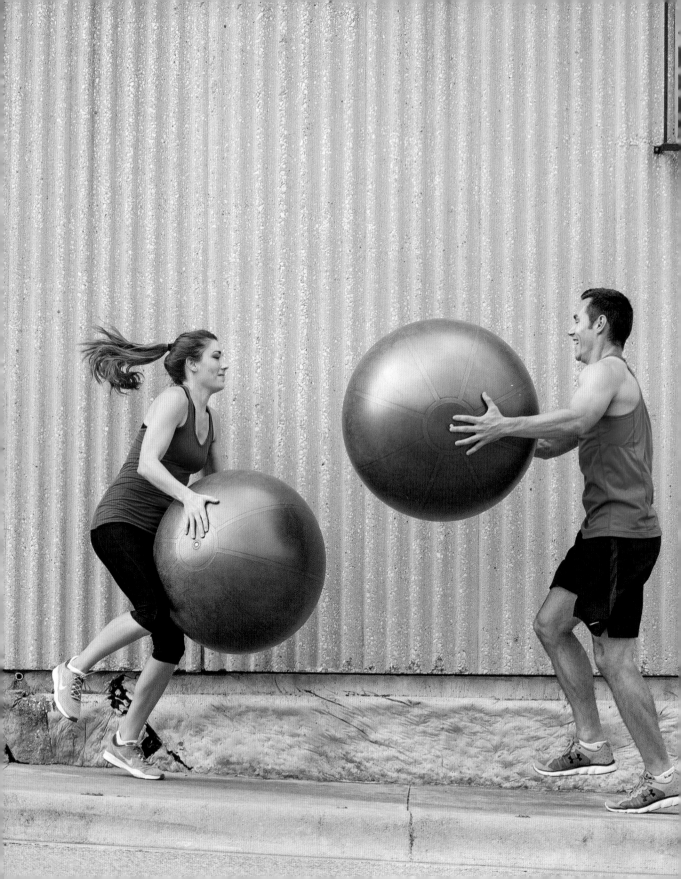

4

STABILITY EXERCISES

These exercises are where your brain and body converge.
You'll test everything from balance and coordination to agility,
flexibility, and reaction time. Despite the wide-ranging style
of exercises that fall into this category, each will help you
enhance your overall neuromotor control.

BOSU REACTION TAPS

REQUIRED EQUIPMENT **BOSU BALL • MEDICINE BALL**

BOSU reaction taps don't just challenge each partner's balance—
they also enhance reaction time, hand-eye coordination, and speed.
Start slowly and pick up the pace as you improve; the faster you go,
the more cardiovascular this exercise becomes.

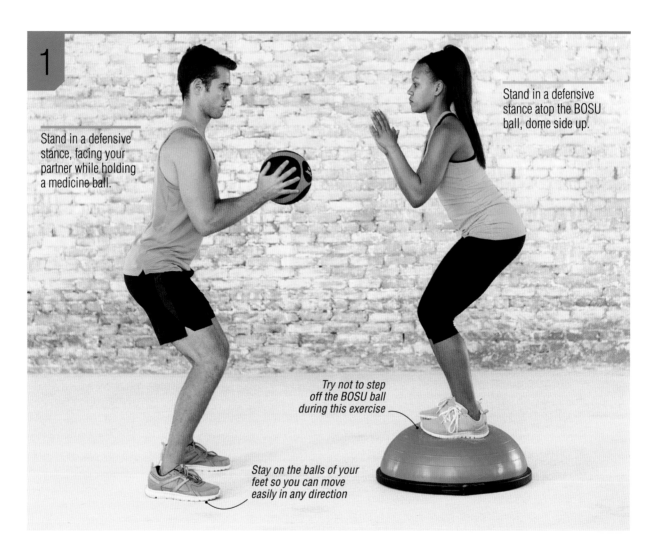

1

Stand in a defensive stance atop the BOSU ball, dome side up.

Stand in a defensive stance, facing your partner while holding a medicine ball.

Try not to step off the BOSU ball during this exercise

Stay on the balls of your feet so you can move easily in any direction

2

Keep the medicine ball in front of you, but move it in unexpected patterns, trying to keep your partner from tapping it.

As your partner moves the medicine ball from spot to spot, try to tap it with both of your hands.

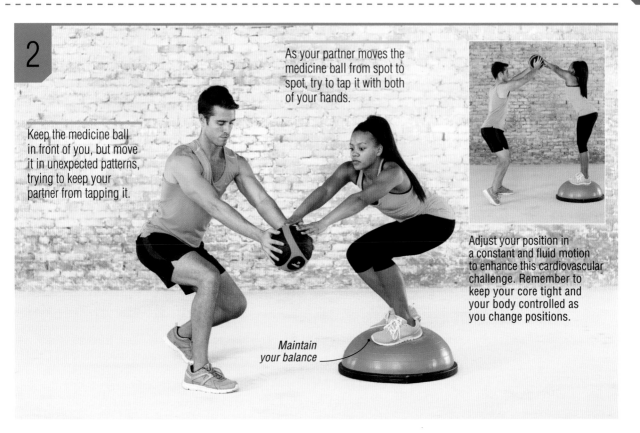

Adjust your position in a constant and fluid motion to enhance this cardiovascular challenge. Remember to keep your core tight and your body controlled as you change positions.

Maintain your balance

3

Change your position often, sliding from side to side, squatting down, or reaching up, as you continue to try to keep your partner from tapping the medicine ball.

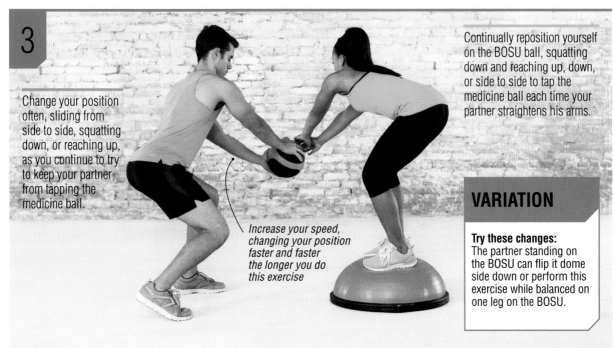

Continually reposition yourself on the BOSU ball, squatting down and reaching up, down, or side to side to tap the medicine ball each time your partner straightens his arms.

Increase your speed, changing your position faster and faster the longer you do this exercise

VARIATION

Try these changes:
The partner standing on the BOSU can flip it dome side down or perform this exercise while balanced on one leg on the BOSU.

DOUBLE DANCER POSE

REQUIRED EQUIPMENT **NONE**

This exercise starts with beginner movements, but the more you challenge yourself to deepen the stretch, the more difficult this exercise becomes. You can expect to test your balance while strengthening your core as well as stretching your quads, hamstrings, hip flexors, chest, and shoulders.

1 Face your partner, reaching forward and pressing your right palm into your partner's right palm. Bend your left knee, lifting your left foot behind you to grasp the top of your left foot with your left hand. Your fingers point up.

MAKE IT
HARDER

You can perform a deeper stretch by bending farther forward from the hips while simultaneously pressing your foot into your palm to lift your legs higher.

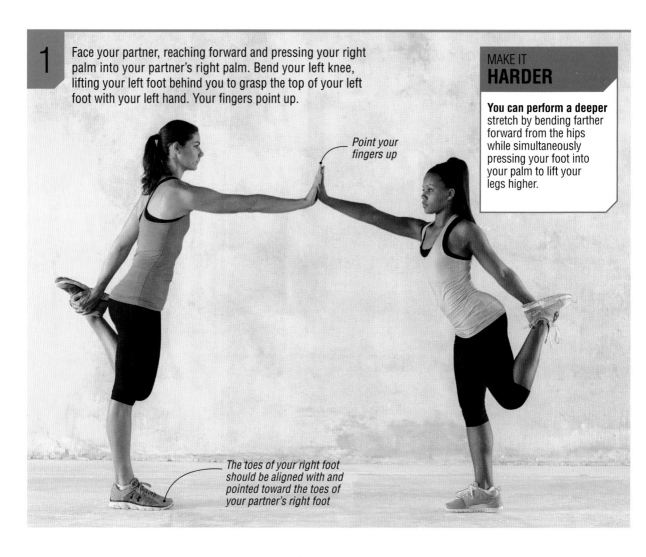

Point your fingers up

The toes of your right foot should be aligned with and pointed toward the toes of your partner's right foot

2 With the muscles of your core contracted, tilt forward from the hips and gradually straighten your right arm upward as you press your left foot into your left hand.

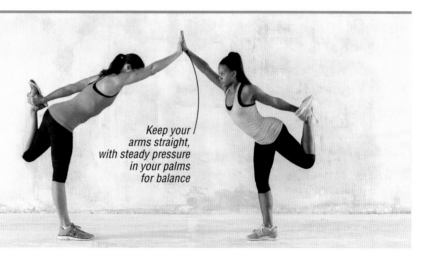

Keep your arms straight, with steady pressure in your palms for balance

3 Tilt farther forward still—as far as your flexibility and balance will allow—keeping your supporting leg straight and using your partner's pressed palm for balance.

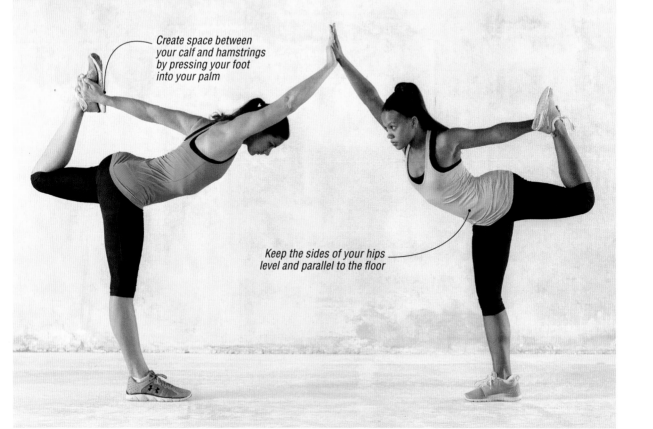

Create space between your calf and hamstrings by pressing your foot into your palm

Keep the sides of your hips level and parallel to the floor

STANDING BACKBEND

REQUIRED EQUIPMENT **NONE**

Stretch your chest, shoulders, and spine as you work with your partner to improve flexibility and balance during this exercise. By using your partner's arms as support, backbends are more accessible and less intimidating than when performed alone.

1 Stand facing your partner, grasping your partner's forearms near her elbows.

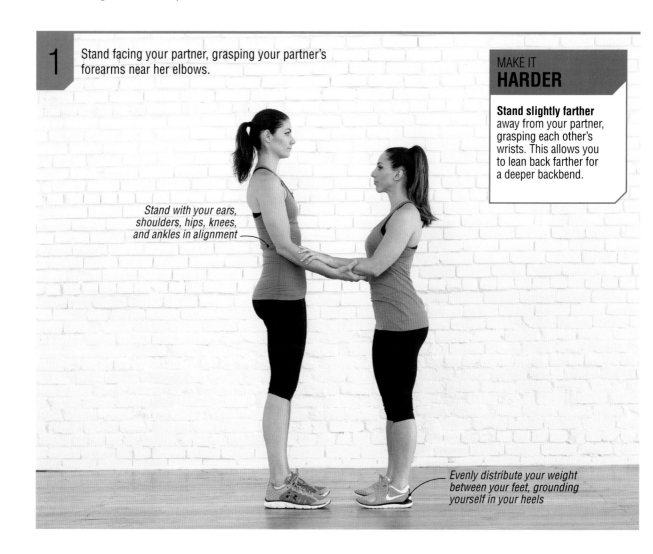

Stand with your ears, shoulders, hips, knees, and ankles in alignment

Evenly distribute your weight between your feet, grounding yourself in your heels

MAKE IT HARDER

Stand slightly farther away from your partner, grasping each other's wrists. This allows you to lean back farther for a deeper backbend.

2 Exhale, lift your chin to look backward, lift your chest to the ceiling, and lean back. Hold this for 3 to 5 deep breaths before returning to an upright position. Repeat this step for the time listed in the workout or as desired.

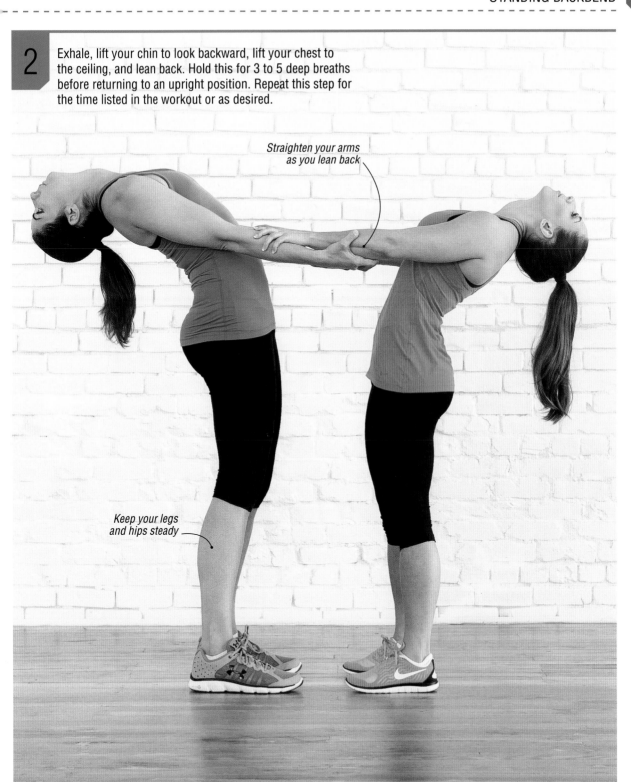

Straighten your arms as you lean back

Keep your legs and hips steady

HAND-SUPPORTED DOUBLE BOAT POSE

REQUIRED EQUIPMENT **NONE**

Fire up your abs, hips, back, and chest as you work on your balance and flexibility with this exercise. Because the double boat has many variations based on ability level, start with this easy version and work your way up to a more challenging pose.

1 Sit facing your partner, bending your knees, with your feet flat on the floor. Start with your toes touching when your knees are bent, but make adjustments as needed, moving closer to or farther away from your partner. Lean back, placing your hands on the floor behind you.

Keep your elbows straight and your chest up

Tighten your abs and lower back

2 Keeping your torso straight, lift your feet off the floor and press them into your partner's feet, maintaining sole-to-sole contact.

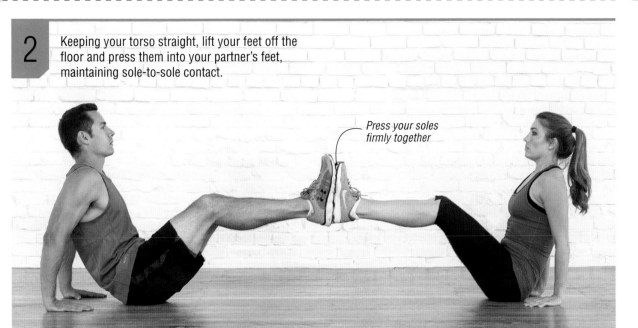

Press your soles firmly together

3 As a unit, try to straighten your legs fully, holding this position for 3 to 5 breaths before returning your feet to the floor. Repeat steps 2 and 3 for the time listed in the workout or as desired.

MAKE IT
HARDER

Start with your hips closer to your partner and turn the pose into an unsupported double boat by reaching forward one hand at a time to grasp your partner's hands.

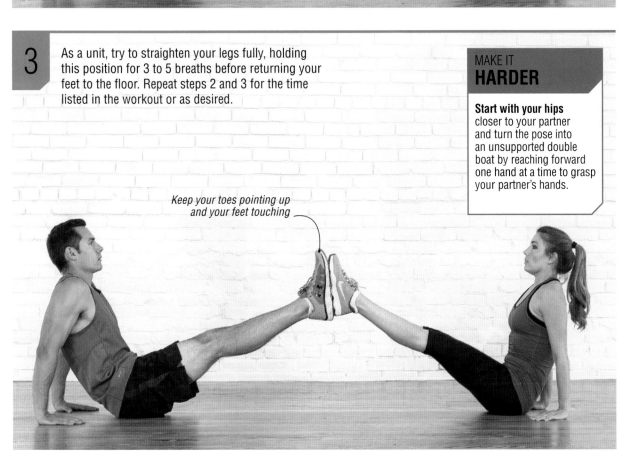

Keep your toes pointing up and your feet touching

CHAIR POSE ON TOES

REQUIRED EQUIPMENT   **NONE**

This static squat exercise is easier to master with the help of your partner's arms for support. The initial phase increases lower-body strength in your glutes and quads, and once you rise up on the balls of your feet, you'll engage your calves while also working on balance.

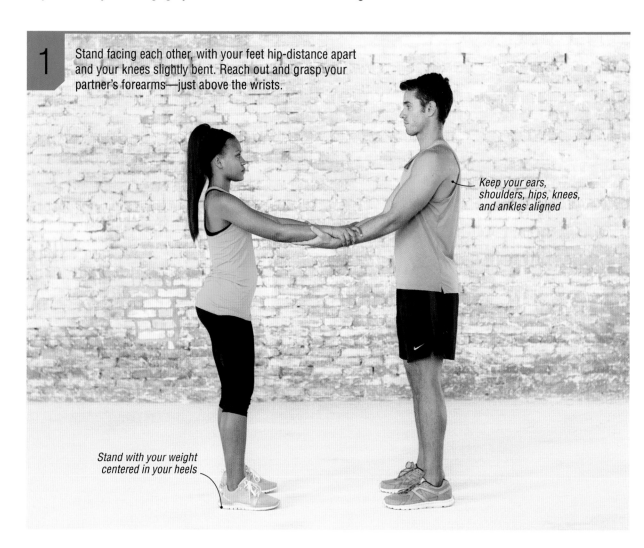

1 Stand facing each other, with your feet hip-distance apart and your knees slightly bent. Reach out and grasp your partner's forearms—just above the wrists.

Keep your ears, shoulders, hips, knees, and ankles aligned

Stand with your weight centered in your heels

2 With your feet flat on the floor and your weight in your heels, engage your hips, abs, and back. Pull your shoulders back to keep your chest lifted, push your hips backward, and bend your knees to lower into a squat.

Look straight ahead at your partner to help keep your chest lifted

Keep your knees aligned with your toes

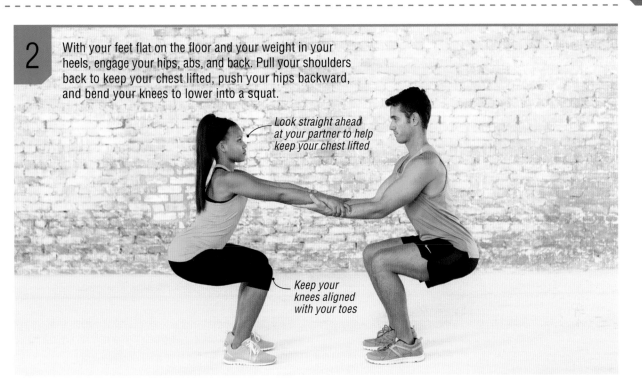

3 Shift your weight forward, lifting your heels off the floor as high as you can. Hold for 3 to 5 breaths, exhale, and repeat steps 2 and 3 for the time listed in the workout or as desired.

Without actually pushing or pulling on your partner, use his arms for support as you lift your heels

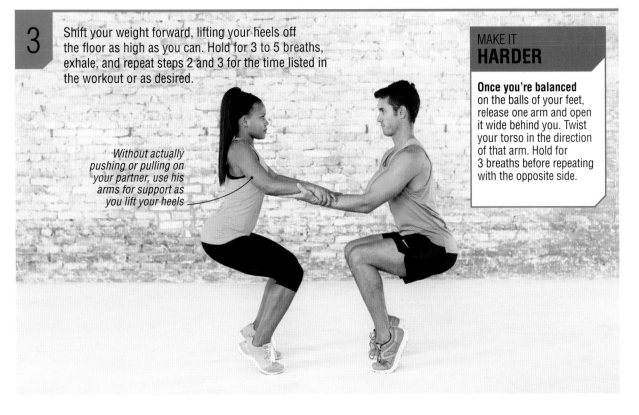

MAKE IT
HARDER

Once you're balanced on the balls of your feet, release one arm and open it wide behind you. Twist your torso in the direction of that arm. Hold for 3 breaths before repeating with the opposite side.

DOUBLE TREE POSE

REQUIRED EQUIPMENT **NONE**

This exercise offers an excellent way to develop single-leg balance because your partner's body helps keep you stabilized while entering the pose. As you progress through this exercise, coordination and core strength from your hips to your shoulders also come into play.

1 Stand side by side with your partner, reaching your inside arm around your partner's waist for support.

2 Pick up your outside foot and bend your knee, rotating your hip outward so your knee swings out to the side and placing the sole of your foot against the inside of your supporting leg.

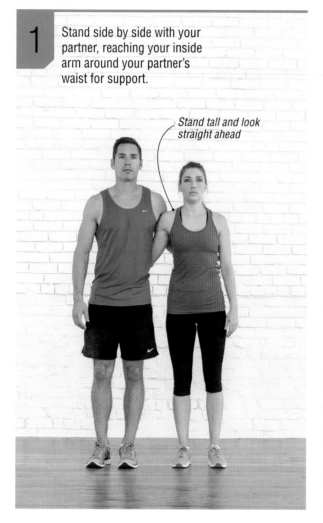

Stand tall and look straight ahead

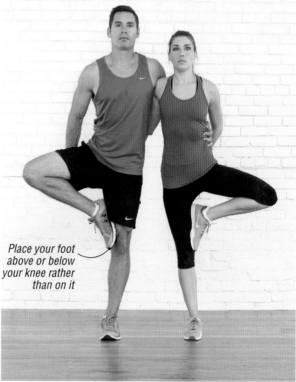

Place your foot above or below your knee rather than on it

3 Press your outer hand against your partner's, palm to palm. Hold for 3 to 5 deep breaths before releasing the pose. Repeat steps 2 and 3 for the time listed in the workout or as desired.

MAKE IT
HARDER

Instead of pressing palms with your partner, grab the toes of your outer foot. Draw your knee up before straightening your leg as much as you can, as if pressing the sole of your outside foot toward the side wall.

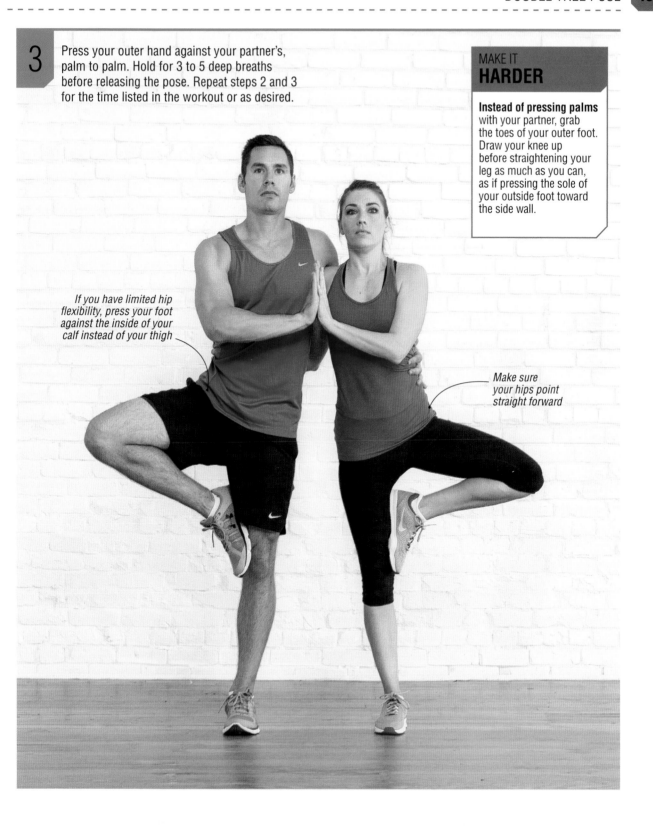

If you have limited hip flexibility, press your foot against the inside of your calf instead of your thigh

Make sure your hips point straight forward

KING OF THE BOSU

REQUIRED EQUIPMENT **MEDICINE BALL • BOSU BALL**

Put the fun back in fitness with this children's game. The goal is to stand on the BOSU ball to maintain your position as king of the BOSU while your partner on the floor tries to throw you off balance. You'll end up working your entire body, but the work will mostly focus on your core.

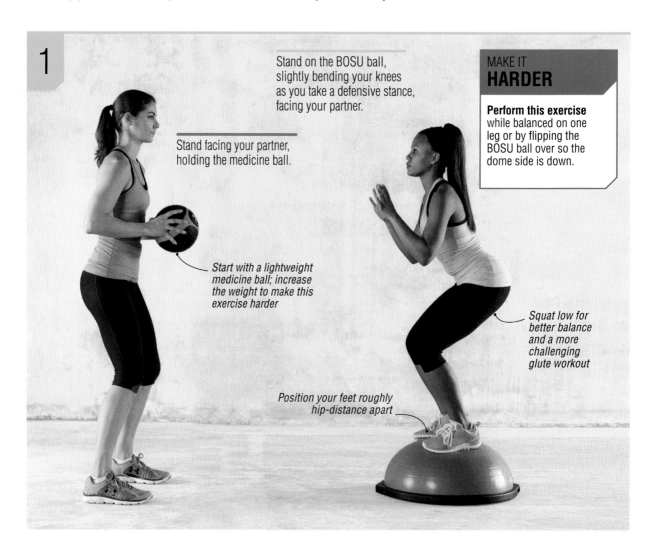

1

Stand on the BOSU ball, slightly bending your knees as you take a defensive stance, facing your partner.

Stand facing your partner, holding the medicine ball.

Start with a lightweight medicine ball; increase the weight to make this exercise harder

Position your feet roughly hip-distance apart

MAKE IT **HARDER**

Perform this exercise while balanced on one leg or by flipping the BOSU ball over so the dome side is down.

Squat low for better balance and a more challenging glute workout

2

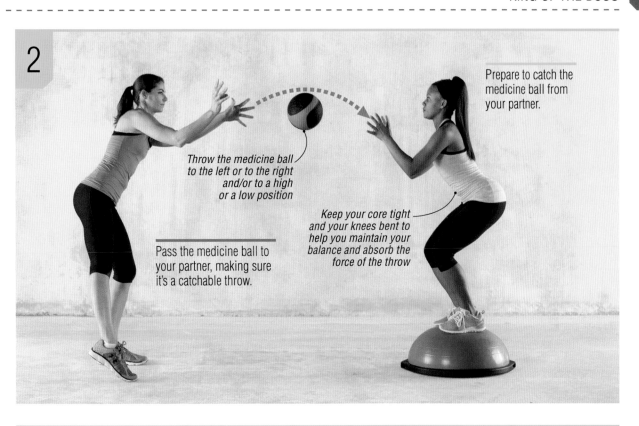

Prepare to catch the medicine ball from your partner.

Throw the medicine ball to the left or to the right and/or to a high or a low position

Keep your core tight and your knees bent to help you maintain your balance and absorb the force of the throw

Pass the medicine ball to your partner, making sure it's a catchable throw.

3

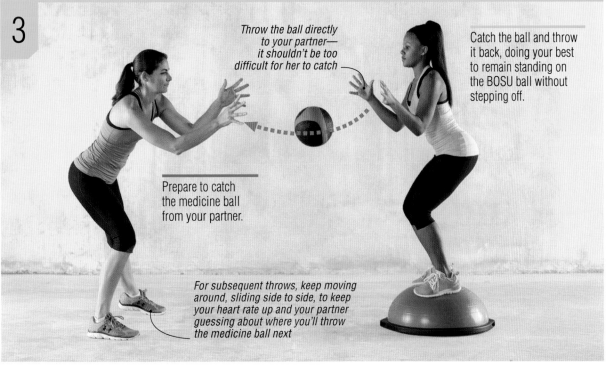

Throw the ball directly to your partner— it shouldn't be too difficult for her to catch

Catch the ball and throw it back, doing your best to remain standing on the BOSU ball without stepping off.

Prepare to catch the medicine ball from your partner.

For subsequent throws, keep moving around, sliding side to side, to keep your heart rate up and your partner guessing about where you'll throw the medicine ball next

PEDALING BOSU V-SIT

REQUIRED EQUIPMENT   **2 BOSU BALLS**

Work your core and hip flexors with this exercise. The trick to performing this movement successfully is working in sync with your partner—communicate constantly, and avoid sudden movements that might knock your partner off her BOSU ball.

1 Place the BOSU balls dome side up, and sit atop your ball while facing your partner, putting your hands on the BOSU for balance. Lean backward slightly to lift your feet, bending your knees to form a V shape with your upper body.

MAKE IT
EASIER

Keep your hands on the BOSU ball to help with your balance.

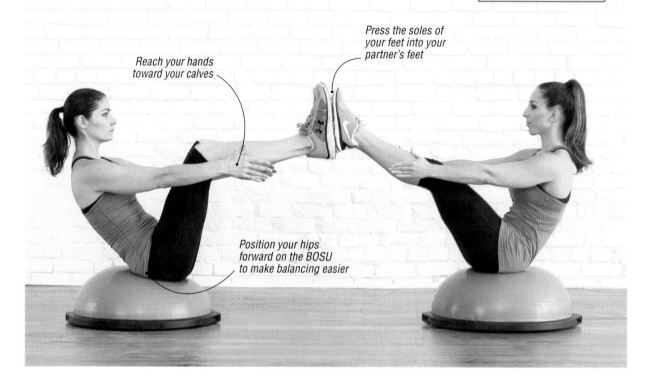

Reach your hands toward your calves

Press the soles of your feet into your partner's feet

Position your hips forward on the BOSU to make balancing easier

2 Move your arms back and forth as you pedal your legs, as if running. Make sure to fully straighten your knees and elbows.

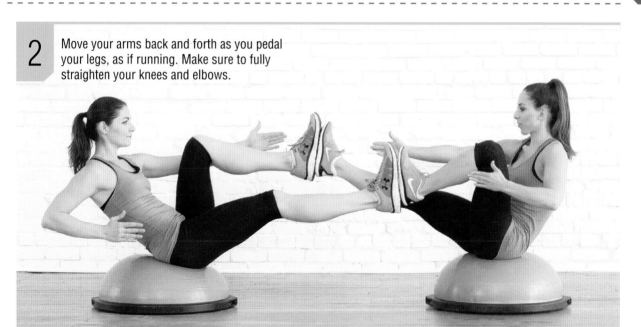

3 Continue to pedal your legs and swing your arms. Repeat steps 2 and 3 for the time listed in the workout or as desired.

MAKE IT
HARDER

Pass a medicine ball back and forth as you pedal your legs.

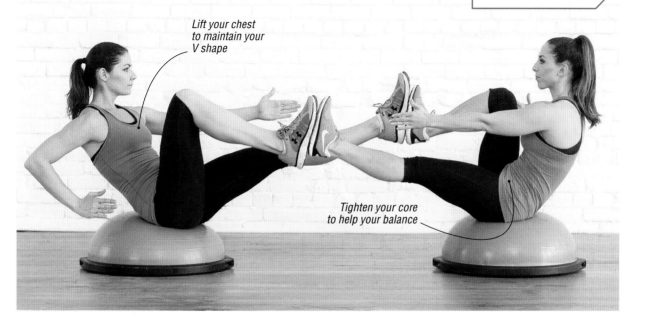

Lift your chest to maintain your V shape

Tighten your core to help your balance

STABILITY BALL PLANK

REQUIRED EQUIPMENT **STABILITY BALL**

Planking on the floor challenges your core, but planking on a stability ball will prove much harder, especially when sharing the stability ball with your partner. Your abs and hips are guaranteed to burn, but don't underestimate the challenge this exercise puts on your shoulders.

1 Kneel on the floor in front of the stability ball, directly across from your partner.

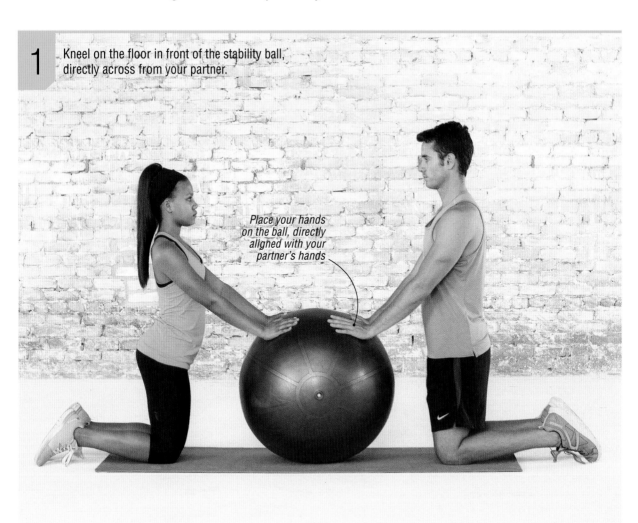

Place your hands on the ball, directly aligned with your partner's hands

2 Lean forward to place your forearms on the stability ball, and with your abs, hips, lower back, and shoulders engaged, find your balance against the ball.

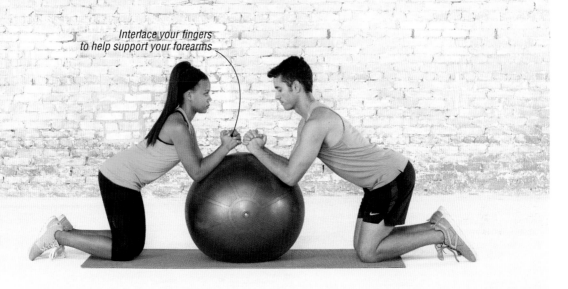

Interlace your fingers to help support your forearms

3 Step your legs—one after the other—behind you, balancing on the balls of your feet and your forearms. Hold your position for the time listed in the workout or as desired.

MAKE IT
HARDER

Place your palms on the stability ball and hold the high plank.

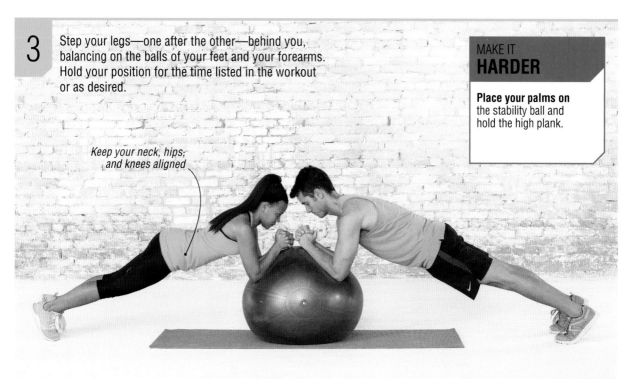

Keep your neck, hips, and knees aligned

WARRIOR III LEG LIFTS

REQUIRED EQUIPMENT **NONE**

Yogis are best known for their flexibility, but many poses, including the Warrior III, offer a significant balance challenge. When performed with a partner, the Warrior III enables you to test your balance limits while simultaneously adding a glute-strengthening leg lift.

1 Stand facing each other, with your right leg holding your weight and your left leg slightly behind you, putting the point of your foot on the floor.

Keep your weight centered over your right heel for better stability

Start with just your toes on the floor

2 Keep your core tight and your back straight as you tip forward from the hips, reaching your arms forward to grasp your partner's upper arms.

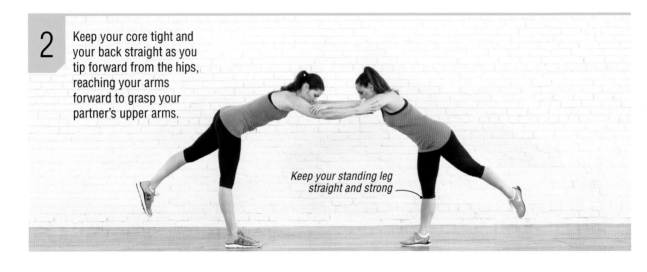

Keep your standing leg straight and strong

3 Tip forward, lifting the back leg so your body forms a T. Lean as far forward as possible so your torso is parallel to the floor.

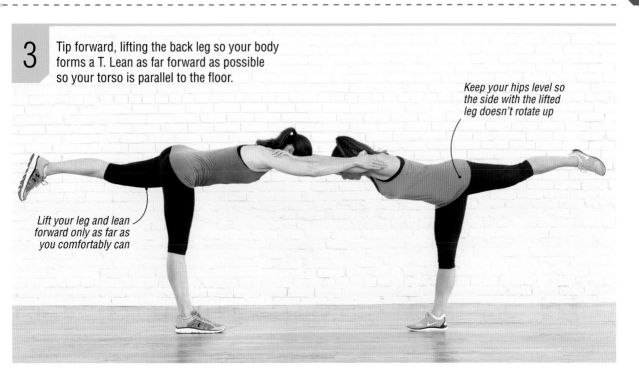

Keep your hips level so the side with the lifted leg doesn't rotate up

Lift your leg and lean forward only as far as you comfortably can

4 Once you're steady, lower your left leg and lift it again as high as you can, tightening the same-side glute. Repeat this step for the time listed in the workout or as desired.

MAKE IT
HARDER

Increase the range of motion of your lifted leg, lowering it until your toes almost touch the floor before lifting it up again.

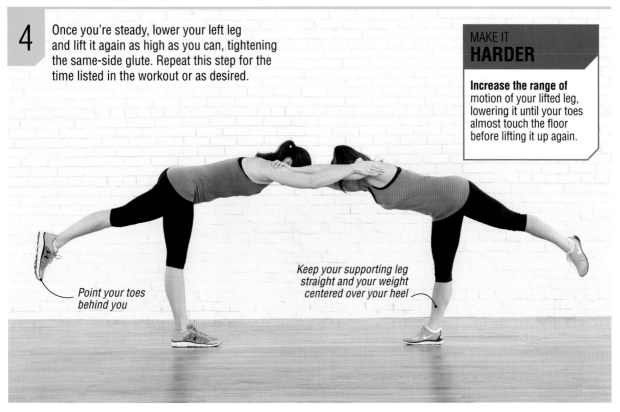

Point your toes behind you

Keep your supporting leg straight and your weight centered over your heel

BOSU
ARM WRESTLING

REQUIRED EQUIPMENT **2 BOSU BALLS**

Arm wrestling might sound like an upper-body activity, but when you do it while balanced on one leg on a BOSU ball, this will become a full-body exercise. Try to beat your partner by forcing him to put his lifted foot down before you do.

1 Stand on top of a BOSU ball, dome side up, facing your partner. Reach out and grasp right hands. Bend your right knee, lifting that leg off the BOSU and suspending it in the air.

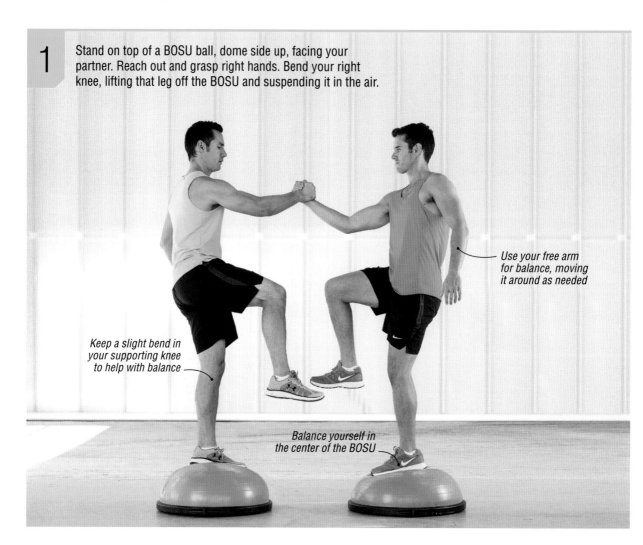

Use your free arm for balance, moving it around as needed

Keep a slight bend in your supporting knee to help with balance

Balance yourself in the center of the BOSU

2 Begin arm wrestling with your partner, using your arm to push his arm away from you to the outside as you both try to maintain balance on one leg.

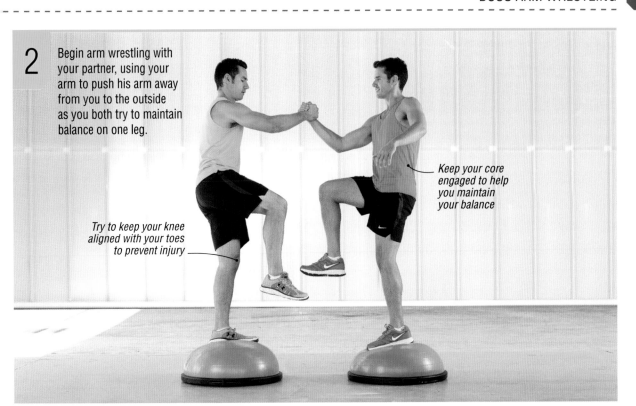

Keep your core engaged to help you maintain your balance

Try to keep your knee aligned with your toes to prevent injury

3 Whenever someone's lifted leg touches the floor, switch arms and feet.

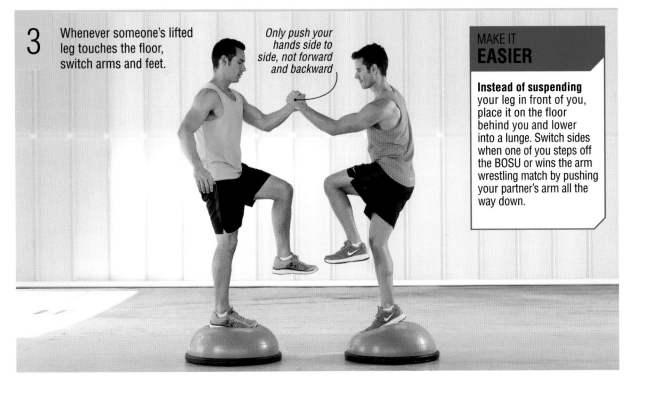

Only push your hands side to side, not forward and backward

MAKE IT
EASIER

Instead of suspending your leg in front of you, place it on the floor behind you and lower into a lunge. Switch sides when one of you steps off the BOSU or wins the arm wrestling match by pushing your partner's arm all the way down.

PUSHING SIDE PLANKS

REQUIRED EQUIPMENT **NONE**

Side planks work your obliques and the rectus abdominis of the core while you hold a static position. This exercise makes the classic side plank more difficult by requiring additional engagement of your hips, lower back, and shoulders as you push against your partner.

1 Kneel on the floor, facing your partner. Lean sideways to place one palm on the floor, mirroring your partner's movements. Straighten your legs, placing one foot on top of the other to enter the side plank position.

MAKE IT EASIER

Bend your top knee, placing your foot on the floor in front of your straightened leg for added support.

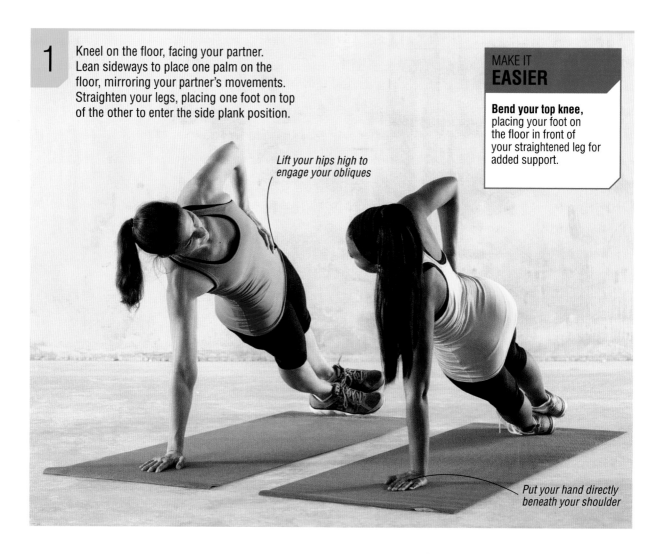

Lift your hips high to engage your obliques

Put your hand directly beneath your shoulder

2 Reach out to grasp your partner's hand. Push and pull against your partner's hand to challenge her balance as you also work on your own balance, trying not to topple over.

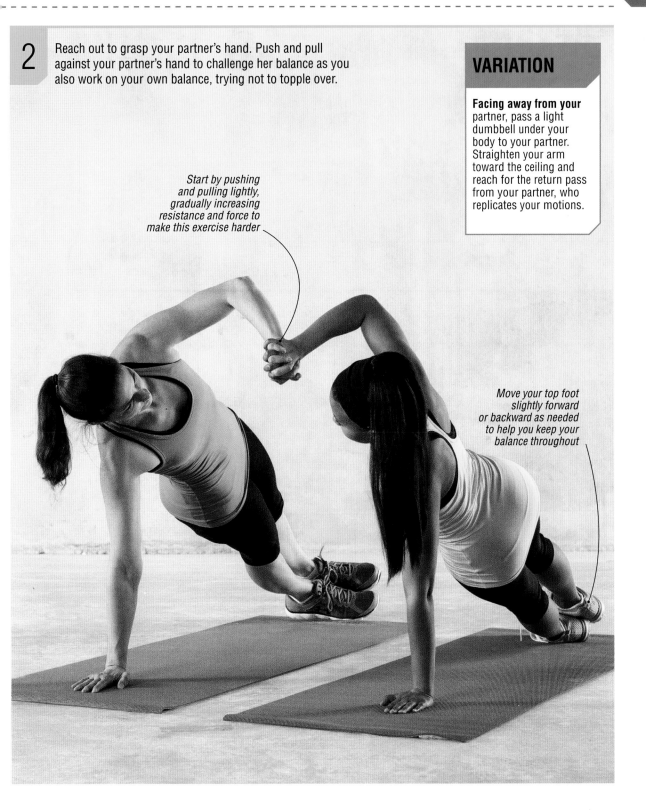

Start by pushing and pulling lightly, gradually increasing resistance and force to make this exercise harder

Move your top foot slightly forward or backward as needed to help you keep your balance throughout

VARIATION

Facing away from your partner, pass a light dumbbell under your body to your partner. Straighten your arm toward the ceiling and reach for the return pass from your partner, who replicates your motions.

DOWNWARD DOG HANDSTAND PIKE

REQUIRED EQUIPMENT **NONE**

This exercise will increase blood flow to your brain while simultaneously stretching your lower body—particularly your hamstrings, glutes, and lower back—and strengthening your upper body, including your shoulders, biceps, and triceps.

1 Start with your hands and knees on the floor. Press your hips up, lift your knees off the floor, and straighten your legs to form an upside down V. This is the downward dog.

Press through your palms, straightening your shoulders and allowing your head to hang between your arms

Stand in front of your partner, facing away, and fold forward from the hips, reaching your hands to the floor, a few inches (centimeters) in front of your partner's hands.

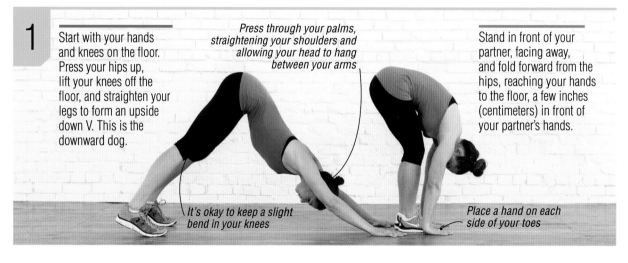

It's okay to keep a slight bend in your knees

Place a hand on each side of your toes

2 Maintain your downward dog position.

Place your toes—one foot at a time—on top of your partner's hips.

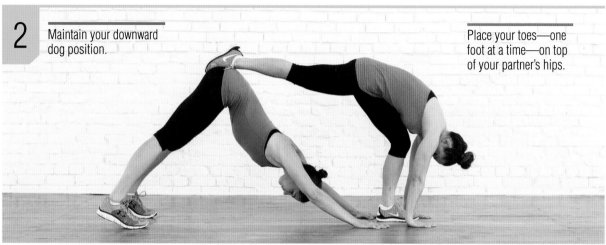

3 Repeat steps 2 and 3 for the time listed in the workout or as desired.

While in the pike position, extend one leg straight up into the air, pointing your toes toward the ceiling. Hold this position for 3 breaths before switching legs.

Press your hips up, pushing through your palms to form a pike. Hold this position for 3 to 5 deep breaths before returning to your starting position.

Straighten your legs, and avoid bending your knees

Maintain your downward dog position.

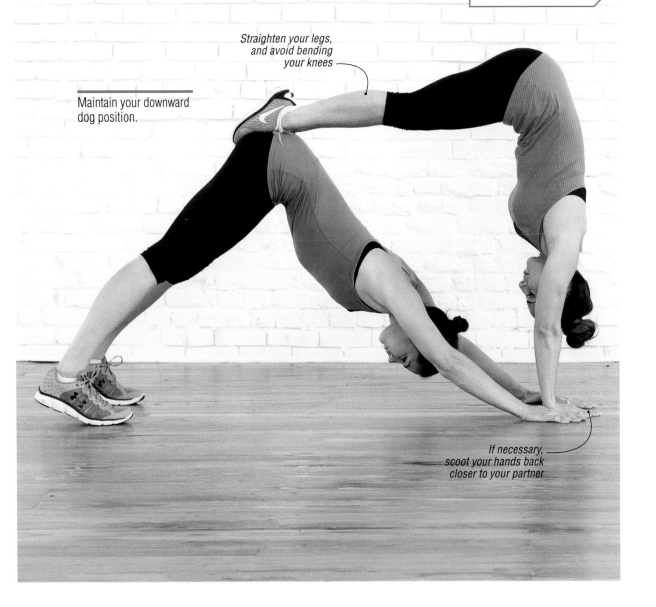

If necessary, scoot your hands back closer to your partner

LEVEL 2

SINGLE-LEG STABILITY BALL BATTLE

REQUIRED EQUIPMENT   **2 STABILITY BALLS**

This exercise will work your core as you try to stay balanced on one leg—all while attempting to force your partner to put a foot on the floor before you do. The harder you work to throw your partner off balance, the greater the cardiovascular challenge will be.

1 Stand facing your partner, holding a stability ball in your hands. Shift your weight to one side, lifting your opposite leg off the floor and bending that knee back.

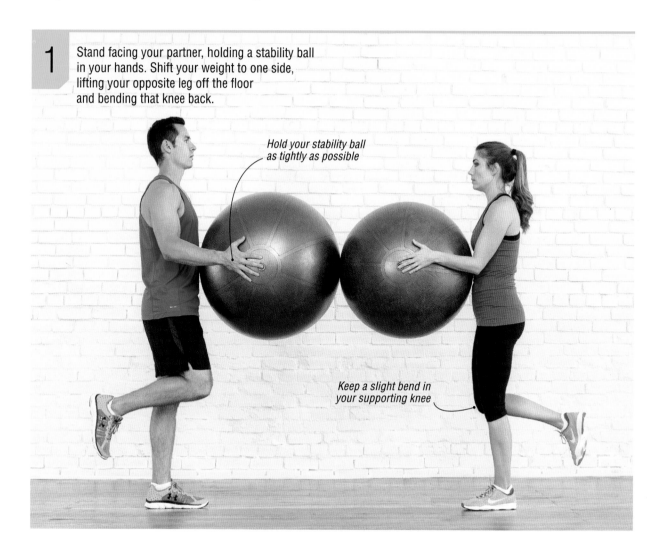

Hold your stability ball as tightly as possible

Keep a slight bend in your supporting knee

2 Use your stability ball to push against your partner's stability ball, trying to force your partner off balance. The goal is to make your partner put his or her lifted foot down before you do.

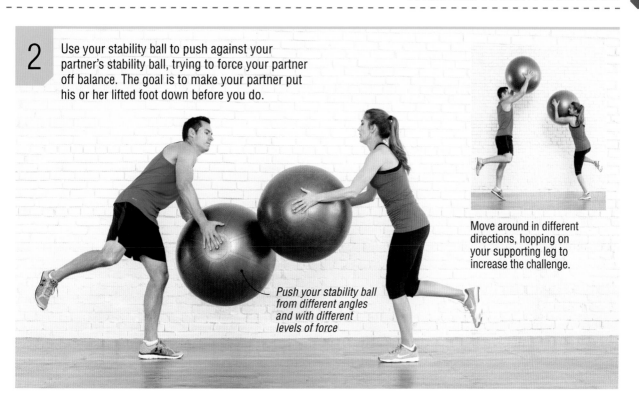

Move around in different directions, hopping on your supporting leg to increase the challenge.

Push your stability ball from different angles and with different levels of force

3 Whenever someone's leg touches down, both partners switch the foot that's suspended in the air before resuming the battle.

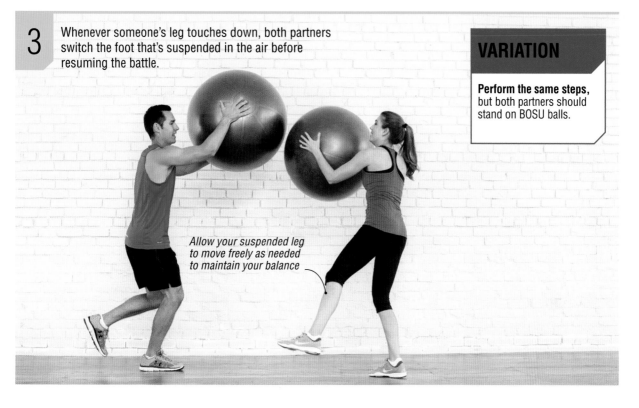

Allow your suspended leg to move freely as needed to maintain your balance

VARIATION

Perform the same steps, but both partners should stand on BOSU balls.

SIDE PLANK & HIP ADDUCTION

REQUIRED EQUIPMENT **NONE**

This exercise will help strengthen your core while targeting your obliques and the adductor muscles of your inner thighs. Protect your lower back by keeping your spine straight. Failing to keep your abs, hips, and lower back contracted and strong has the potential for injury.

1

Start in side plank, with one palm on the floor directly under your shoulder, stacking your feet so your body forms a straight line from the center of your forehead to the midline between your feet.

MAKE IT **EASIER**

Perform the side plank with your elbow bent. You can also bend your lower leg at the knee, making the hip adduction easier. Allow your partner to lift your top leg.

Keep your body in this straight line, lifting your top hip when your partner lifts your leg up

Straddle your partner's legs, squat down to grasp your partner's top leg with both hands, and return to standing, holding your partner's leg between your own.

Start in a defensive stance, tightening your shoulders, lower back, abs, and hips to engage your core

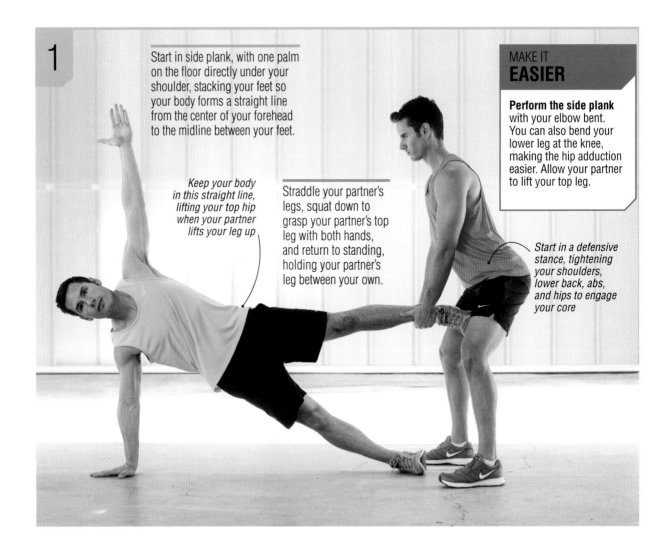

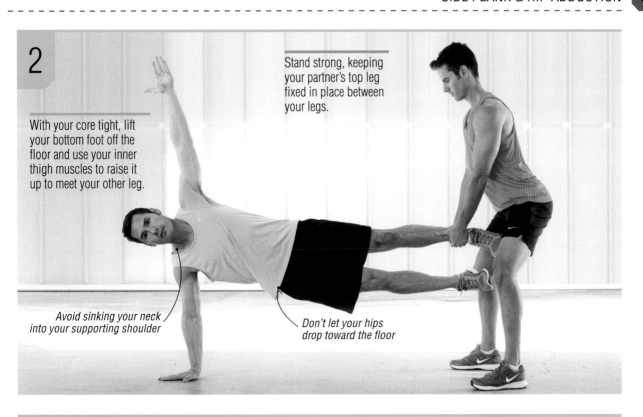

2

With your core tight, lift your bottom foot off the floor and use your inner thigh muscles to raise it up to meet your other leg.

Stand strong, keeping your partner's top leg fixed in place between your legs.

Avoid sinking your neck into your supporting shoulder

Don't let your hips drop toward the floor

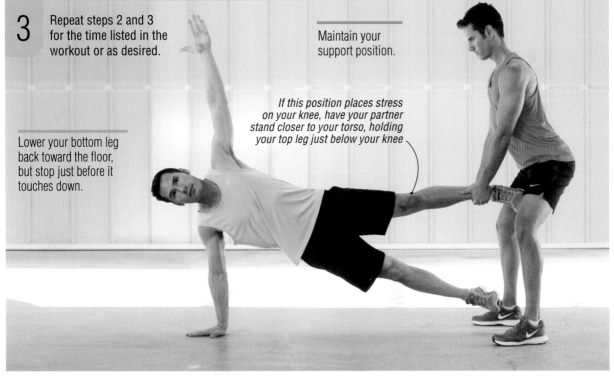

3

Repeat steps 2 and 3 for the time listed in the workout or as desired.

Maintain your support position.

If this position places stress on your knee, have your partner stand closer to your torso, holding your top leg just below your knee

Lower your bottom leg back toward the floor, but stop just before it touches down.

STACKED PLANK

REQUIRED EQUIPMENT **NONE**

This is an acrobatic, yoga-inspired move that requires you to engage your entire body—shoulders, chest, triceps, back, abdominals, glutes, and quads—while holding a static plank. One partner isn't simply supporting her own weight—she's also supporting her partner's weight.

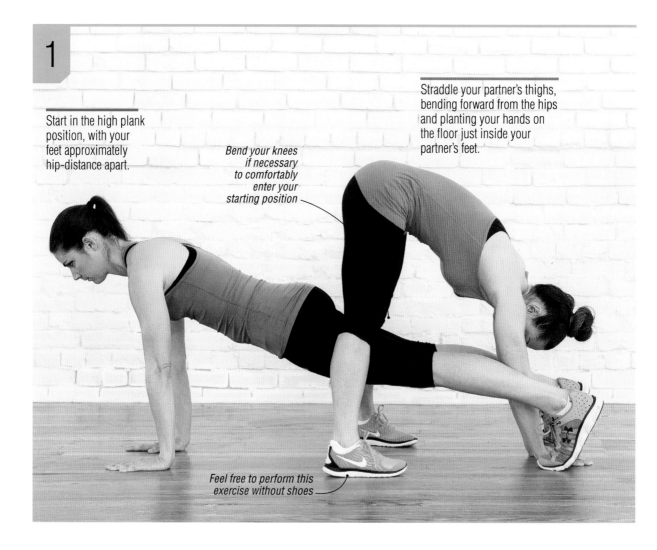

1

Start in the high plank position, with your feet approximately hip-distance apart.

Bend your knees if necessary to comfortably enter your starting position

Straddle your partner's thighs, bending forward from the hips and planting your hands on the floor just inside your partner's feet.

Feel free to perform this exercise without shoes

2

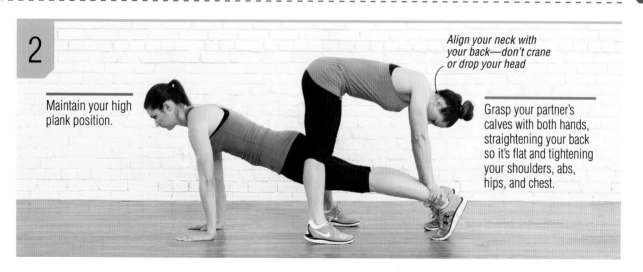

Maintain your high plank position.

Align your neck with your back—don't crane or drop your head

Grasp your partner's calves with both hands, straightening your back so it's flat and tightening your shoulders, abs, hips, and chest.

3

Continue to maintain your high plank, tightening your core to prepare to take on your partner's weight.

Lift each leg one at a time, placing the ball of one foot and then the other onto your partner's shoulders to enter into the high plank position.

VARIATION

Recruit a third partner to add an additional plank. The third partner places his hands on the calves of the second partner and then places his feet across the second partner's shoulders to enter into the high plank.

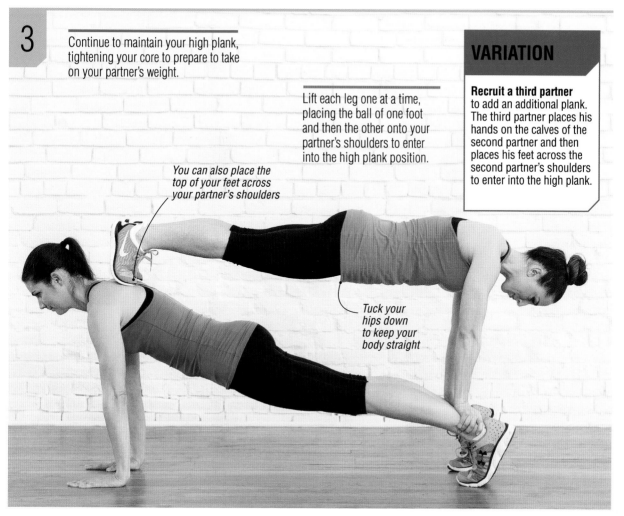

You can also place the top of your feet across your partner's shoulders

Tuck your hips down to keep your body straight

KNEELING BALANCE & PASS

REQUIRED EQUIPMENT **MEDICINE BALL • STABILITY BALL**

This exercise requires exceptional core strength and balance as you focus on staying atop a stability ball while catching your partner's medicine ball passes. Engage your core while keeping your upper body loose—avoid tensing your neck, shoulders, or upper back.

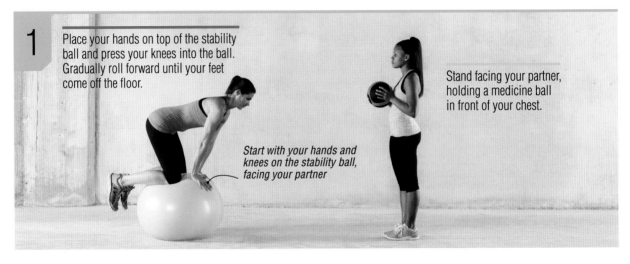

1 Place your hands on top of the stability ball and press your knees into the ball. Gradually roll forward until your feet come off the floor.

Start with your hands and knees on the stability ball, facing your partner

Stand facing your partner, holding a medicine ball in front of your chest.

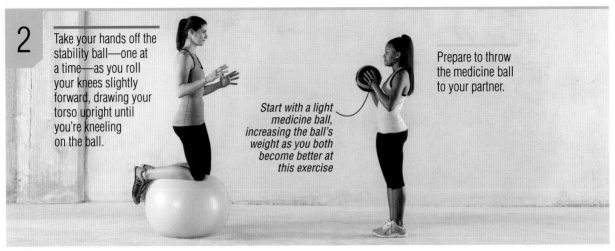

2 Take your hands off the stability ball—one at a time—as you roll your knees slightly forward, drawing your torso upright until you're kneeling on the ball.

Start with a light medicine ball, increasing the ball's weight as you both become better at this exercise

Prepare to throw the medicine ball to your partner.

3

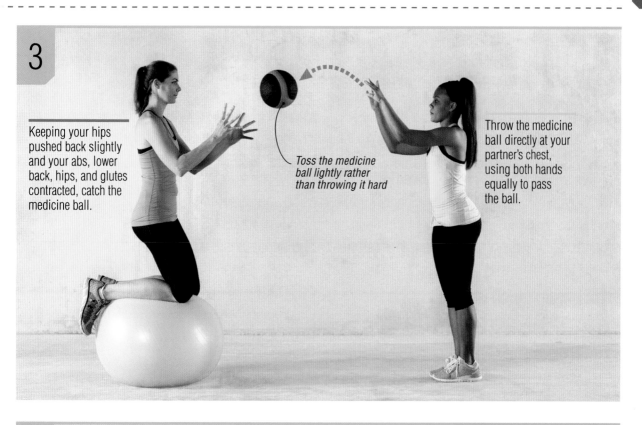

Keeping your hips pushed back slightly and your abs, lower back, hips, and glutes contracted, catch the medicine ball.

Toss the medicine ball lightly rather than throwing it hard

Throw the medicine ball directly at your partner's chest, using both hands equally to pass the ball.

4

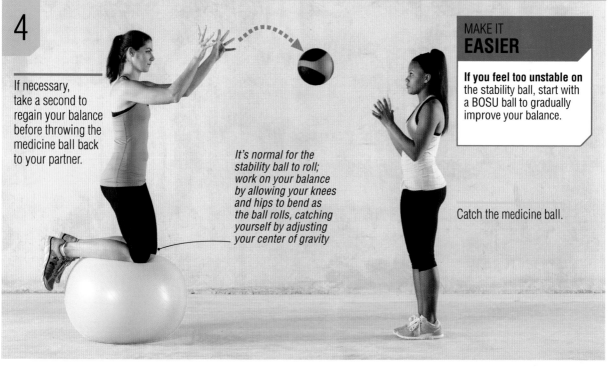

If necessary, take a second to regain your balance before throwing the medicine ball back to your partner.

It's normal for the stability ball to roll; work on your balance by allowing your knees and hips to bend as the ball rolls, catching yourself by adjusting your center of gravity

MAKE IT
EASIER

If you feel too unstable on the stability ball, start with a BOSU ball to gradually improve your balance.

Catch the medicine ball.

STABILITY BALL BALANCE & JAB

REQUIRED EQUIPMENT **STABILITY BALL • BOSU BALL**

For this exercise, when you're jabbing, you'll develop core strength in your glutes, hips, abs, and shoulders while increasing your heart rate for a burst of cardio. This type of intermittent cardio during a training session is an excellent way to improve heart health and endurance.

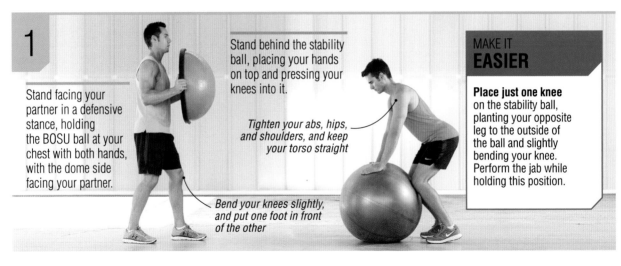

1

Stand facing your partner in a defensive stance, holding the BOSU ball at your chest with both hands, with the dome side facing your partner.

Stand behind the stability ball, placing your hands on top and pressing your knees into it.

Tighten your abs, hips, and shoulders, and keep your torso straight

Bend your knees slightly, and put one foot in front of the other

MAKE IT EASIER

Place just one knee on the stability ball, planting your opposite leg to the outside of the ball and slightly bending your knee. Perform the jab while holding this position.

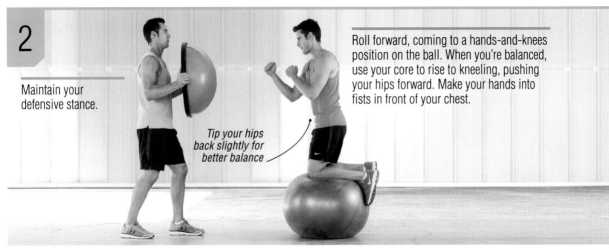

2

Maintain your defensive stance.

Roll forward, coming to a hands-and-knees position on the ball. When you're balanced, use your core to rise to kneeling, pushing your hips forward. Make your hands into fists in front of your chest.

Tip your hips back slightly for better balance

3

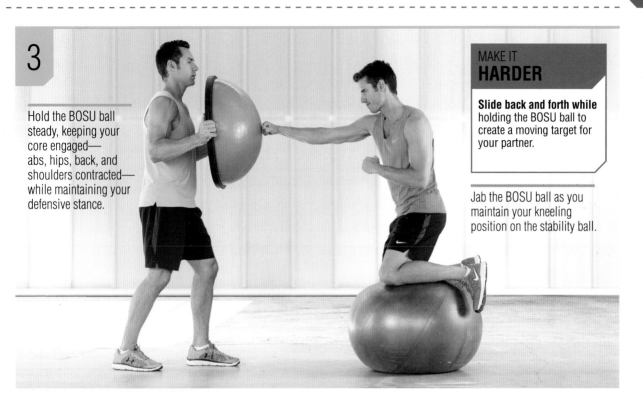

Hold the BOSU ball steady, keeping your core engaged—abs, hips, back, and shoulders contracted—while maintaining your defensive stance.

MAKE IT
HARDER

Slide back and forth while holding the BOSU ball to create a moving target for your partner.

Jab the BOSU ball as you maintain your kneeling position on the stability ball.

4

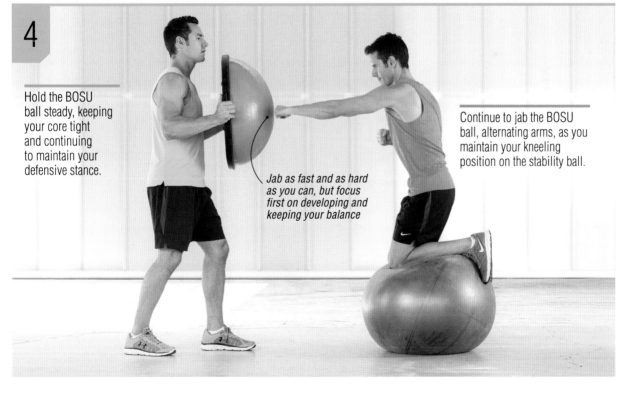

Hold the BOSU ball steady, keeping your core tight and continuing to maintain your defensive stance.

Jab as fast and as hard as you can, but focus first on developing and keeping your balance

Continue to jab the BOSU ball, alternating arms, as you maintain your kneeling position on the stability ball.

FLYING BIRD POSE

REQUIRED EQUIPMENT   **NONE**

This acrobatic, yoga-inspired pose is much like a plank, but instead of balancing on your hands and the balls of your feet, you'll balance on your partner's straightened legs. Keep the muscles of your entire body—from your shoulders to your calves—engaged for support.

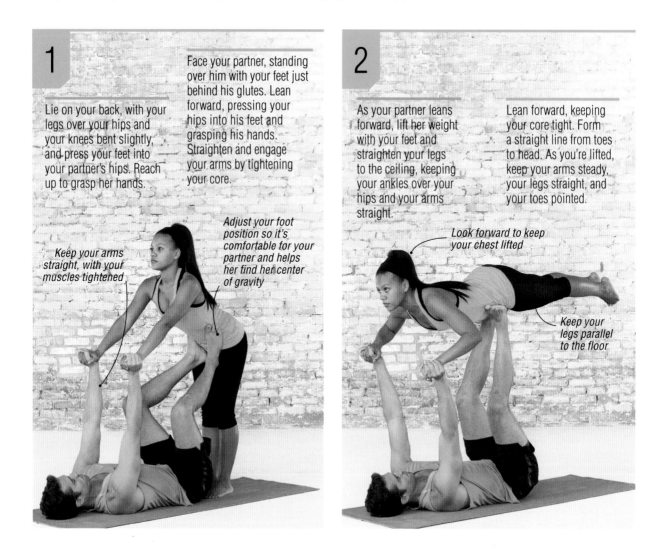

1

Lie on your back, with your legs over your hips and your knees bent slightly, and press your feet into your partner's hips. Reach up to grasp her hands.

Face your partner, standing over him with your feet just behind his glutes. Lean forward, pressing your hips into his feet and grasping his hands. Straighten and engage your arms by tightening your core.

Keep your arms straight, with your muscles tightened

Adjust your foot position so it's comfortable for your partner and helps her find her center of gravity

2

As your partner leans forward, lift her weight with your feet and straighten your legs to the ceiling, keeping your ankles over your hips and your arms straight.

Lean forward, keeping your core tight. Form a straight line from toes to head. As you're lifted, keep your arms steady, your legs straight, and your toes pointed.

Look forward to keep your chest lifted

Keep your legs parallel to the floor

3 Hold this position for 10 seconds or as long as you can. Breathe slowly. Once you're balanced (and only if you're comfortable with doing so), release your grip on each other—one hand at a time.

MAKE IT
HARDER
The partner in the air points her arms toward her toes instead of to the side.

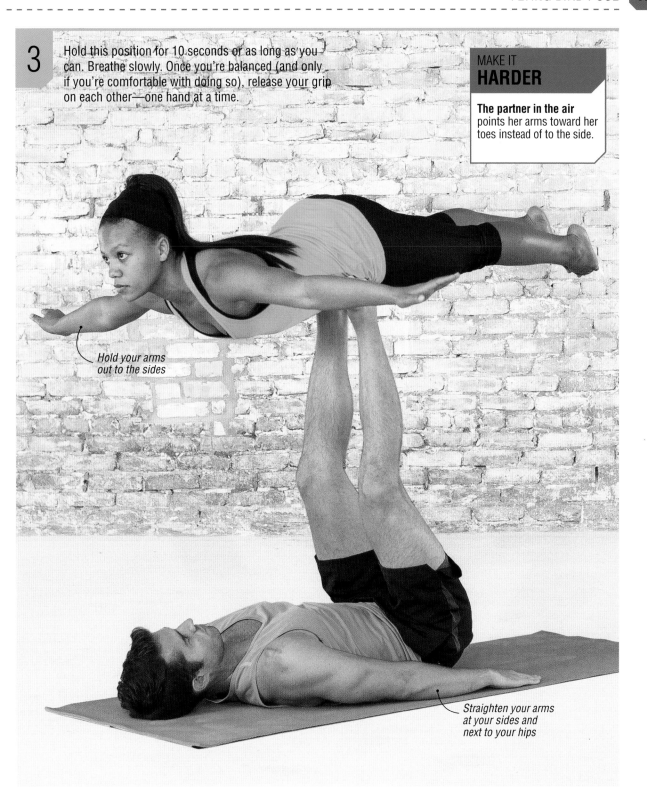

Hold your arms
out to the sides

Straighten your arms
at your sides and
next to your hips

BOSU BALL BATTLE

REQUIRED EQUIPMENT   **STABILITY BALL • BOSU BALL**

Having a ball battle on a BOSU looks relatively easy, but it requires significant balance and core strength to maintain your footing. Performing this and other balance exercises regularly will enhance your core strength, coordination, and how your body reacts to stimuli.

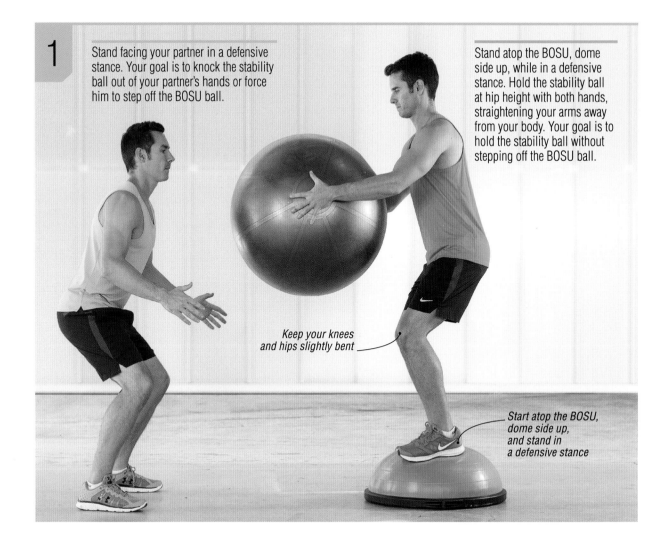

1 Stand facing your partner in a defensive stance. Your goal is to knock the stability ball out of your partner's hands or force him to step off the BOSU ball.

Stand atop the BOSU, dome side up, while in a defensive stance. Hold the stability ball at hip height with both hands, straightening your arms away from your body. Your goal is to hold the stability ball without stepping off the BOSU ball.

Keep your knees and hips slightly bent

Start atop the BOSU, dome side up, and stand in a defensive stance

2

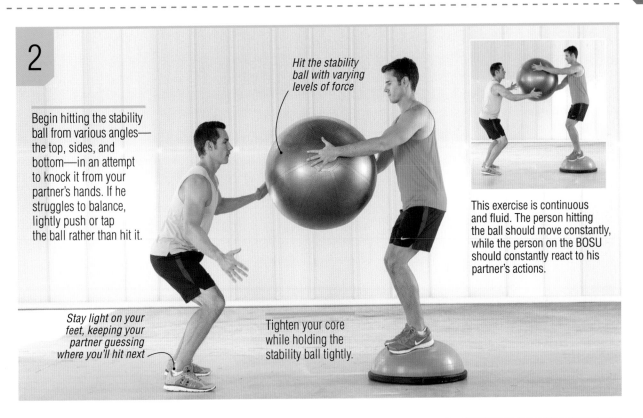

Begin hitting the stability ball from various angles—the top, sides, and bottom—in an attempt to knock it from your partner's hands. If he struggles to balance, lightly push or tap the ball rather than hit it.

Hit the stability ball with varying levels of force

This exercise is continuous and fluid. The person hitting the ball should move constantly, while the person on the BOSU should constantly react to his partner's actions.

Stay light on your feet, keeping your partner guessing where you'll hit next

Tighten your core while holding the stability ball tightly.

3

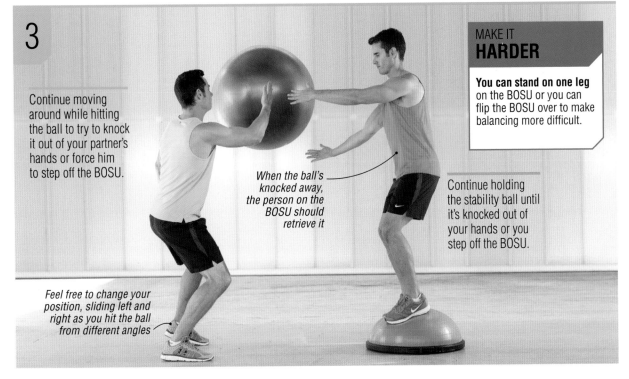

Continue moving around while hitting the ball to try to knock it out of your partner's hands or force him to step off the BOSU.

When the ball's knocked away, the person on the BOSU should retrieve it

MAKE IT
HARDER

You can stand on one leg on the BOSU or you can flip the BOSU over to make balancing more difficult.

Continue holding the stability ball until it's knocked out of your hands or you step off the BOSU.

Feel free to change your position, sliding left and right as you hit the ball from different angles

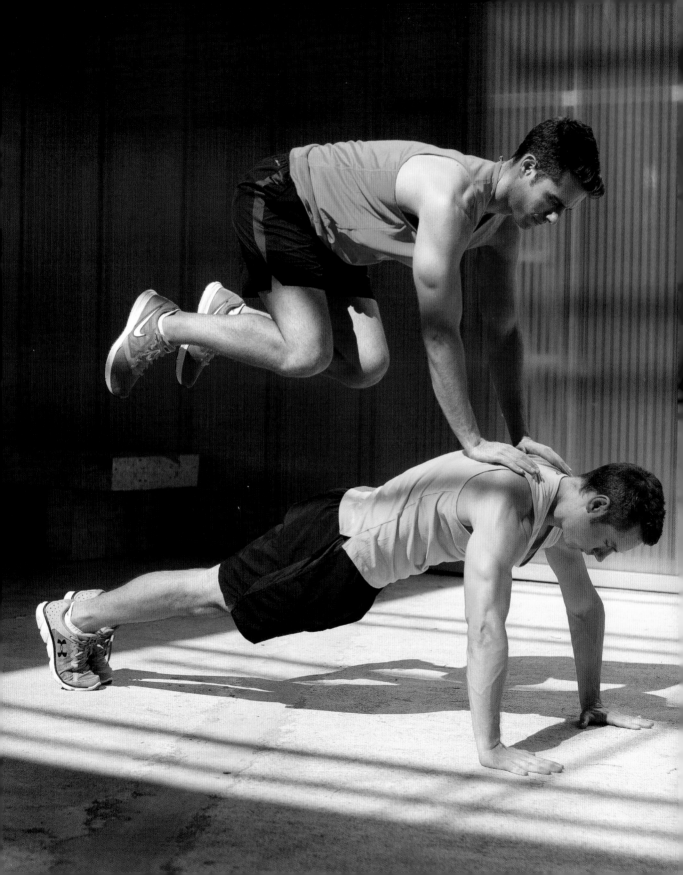

5

PROGRAMS
& WORKOUTS

It's good to master an exercise, better to master a workout,
and better still to complete a full workout program. Lucky for you,
all three options are available. Simply grab your favorite partner
and choose the workout or program that's best suited to your
ability level—and work toward reaching your fitness goals.

LEVEL 1 PROGRAM

The workouts in this program are for beginners, but because partners sometimes progress at different speeds or start a program at different levels, these workouts are adaptive and progressive, becoming more difficult as the weeks pass.

WEEK 1

DAY	WORKOUT	PAGE
1	Short Circuits	187
2	Rest	
3	Circ-HIIT	187
4	Rest	
5	Rest	
6	Strike a Balance	188
7	Rest	

WEEK 2

DAY	WORKOUT	PAGE
1	Short Circuits	187
2	Rest	
3	Strike a Balance	188
4	Rest	
5	Circ-HIIT	187
6	Lower-Body Burner and Core Blitz	191 and 192
7	Rest	

WEEK 3

DAY	WORKOUT	PAGE
1	Upper-Body Burner and Core Blitz	192
2	4x4 Challenge	189
3	Rest	
4	Rest	
5	Upper-Body Burner and Core Blitz	192
6	4x4 Challenge	188
7	Rest	

WEEK 4

DAY	WORKOUT	PAGE
1	Come on Strong	195
2	Cellular Excitation and Core Blitz	195 and 192
3	Rest	
4	Rest	
5	Twisted Tabata and Lower-Body Burner	191
6	Come on Strong	195
7	Rest	

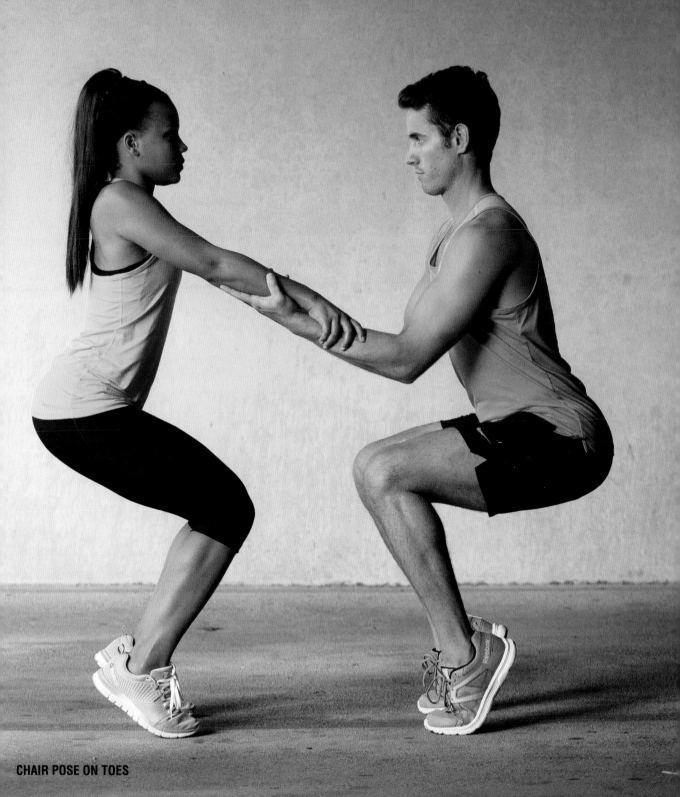

CHAIR POSE ON TOES

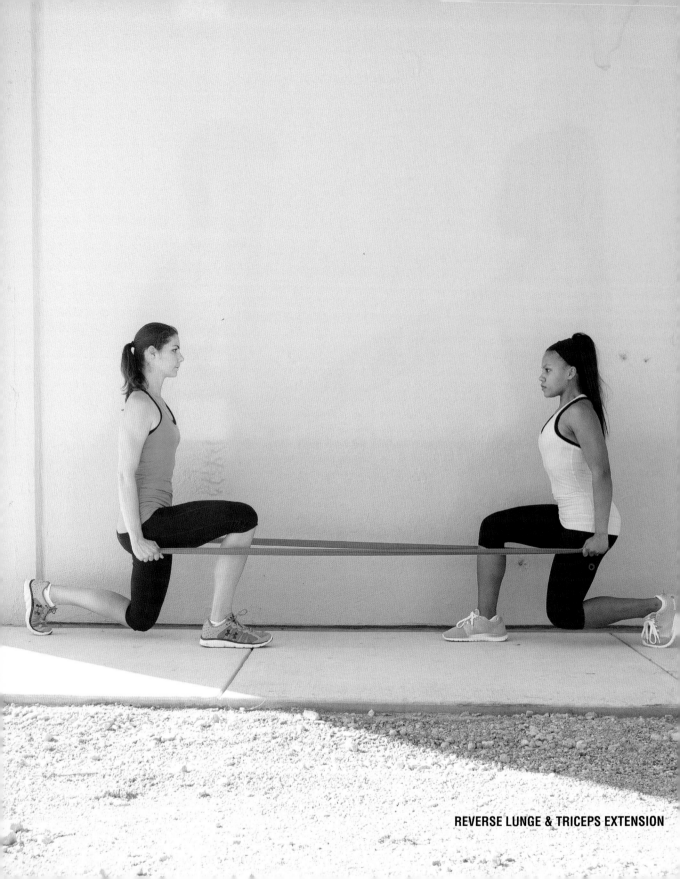

REVERSE LUNGE & TRICEPS EXTENSION

LEVEL 1

SHORT CIRCUITS

Circuit training is perfect for partner workouts because it ensures both partners stay active, boosting their heart rates while cycling through each series of exercises.

YOU'LL NEED

Timer	2 resistance bands
Medicine ball	BOSU ball

CIRCUIT 1

EXERCISE	TIME	REST	PAGE
Squat, Reach & Pass	60 secs		50
Sliding Chest Pass	60 secs		54
Reverse Lunge & Triceps Extension	60 secs	30 secs	42

Perform 3 times total, alternating roles with your partner each round.

CIRCUIT 2

EXERCISE	TIME	REST	PAGE
Resistance Band Chest Press & Row	60 secs		48
Superman Lats & Biceps Curls	60 secs		40
Resisted Shoulder Press	60 secs	30 secs	90

Perform 4 times total, alternating roles with your partner each round.

CIRCUIT 3

EXERCISE	TIME	REST	PAGE
BOSU Reaction Taps	60 secs		142
Side Lunge & Twist	60 secs		38
Chair Pose on Toes	30 secs	30 secs	150

Perform 2 times total, alternating roles with your partner each round.

CIRC-HIIT

This HIIT (high-intensity interval training) variation combines bursts of high-intensity cardio with more low-key strength training designed to keep your heart rate elevated.

YOU'LL NEED

Timer	Medicine ball
2 resistance bands	Stability ball

CIRCUIT 1

EXERCISE	TIME	REST	PAGE
Squat & Resistance Band Sprint	50 secs	10 secs	36
Squat & Resistance Band Sprint (switch roles)	50 secs	10 secs	36
Bear Crawl & Static Row	50 secs	10 secs	58
Bear Crawl & Static Row (switch roles)	50 secs	60 secs	58

Perform 4 times total, alternating roles as instructed.

CIRCUIT 2

EXERCISE	TIME	REST	PAGE
Reverse Lunge & Triceps Extension	50 secs	10 secs	42
Resistance Band Chest Press & Row	50 secs	10 secs	48
Resistance Band Chest Press & Row (switch roles)	50 secs	60 secs	48

Perform 4 times total, alternating roles as instructed.

CIRCUIT 3

EXERCISE	TIME	REST	PAGE
Sliding Chest Pass	50 secs	10 secs	54
Back-to-Back Squats	50 secs	10 secs	88
Lateral Medicine Ball Toss	50 secs	10 secs	60
Stability Ball Situp & Pass	50 secs	60 secs	52

Perform 4 times total, alternating roles after each round.

LEVEL 1

STRIKE A BALANCE

This workout's real demand comes as a balance challenge. Every other move is a stability-training exercise. Use this to slow your breathing and focus on whole-body equilibrium.

YOU'LL NEED

Timer
2 medicine balls

CIRCUIT

EXERCISE	TIME	REST	PAGE
Squat, Reach & Pass	60 secs		50
Chair Pose on Toes	60 secs		150
Wheelbarrow Walk	60 secs		96
Standing Backbend	60 secs		146
Alternating Getup	60 secs		102
Hand-Supported Double Boat Pose	60 secs		148
Coordinated Lunges	60 secs		92
Double Dancer Pose	60 secs		144
Unstable Pushup & Medicine Ball Roll	60 secs		62
Warrior III Leg Lifts	60 secs	60 secs	160

Perform 4 times total, alternating roles after each round as needed.

4X4 CHALLENGE

This offers four exercises per circuit designed to target your upper body, lower body, and core. The challenge comes from performing the routine four times in a row.

YOU'LL NEED

Timer
2 resistance bands
Dumbbell
Stability ball

CIRCUIT 1

EXERCISE	TIME	REST	PAGE
Squat & Resistance Band Sprint	50 secs	10 secs	36
Weighted Plank & Dumbbell Row	50 secs	10 secs	44
Resisted Shoulder Press	50 secs	10 secs	90
Leg Throws	50 secs	60 secs	70

CIRCUIT 2

EXERCISE	TIME	REST	PAGE
Side Lunge & Twist	50 secs	10 secs	38
Weighted Plank & Triceps Extension	50 secs	10 secs	46
Superman Lats & Biceps Curls	50 secs	10 secs	40
Stability Ball Situp & Pass	50 secs	60 secs	52

CIRCUIT 3

EXERCISE	TIME	REST	PAGE
Reverse Lunge & Triceps Extension	50 secs	10 secs	42
Resistance Band Chest Press & Row	50 secs	10 secs	48
Plank & Bridge	50 secs	10 secs	110
Hand-Supported Double Boat Pose	50 secs	60 secs	148

Once you've completed the third circuit, perform the whole routine three more times. Switch roles with your partner where appropriate each time you perform the workout.

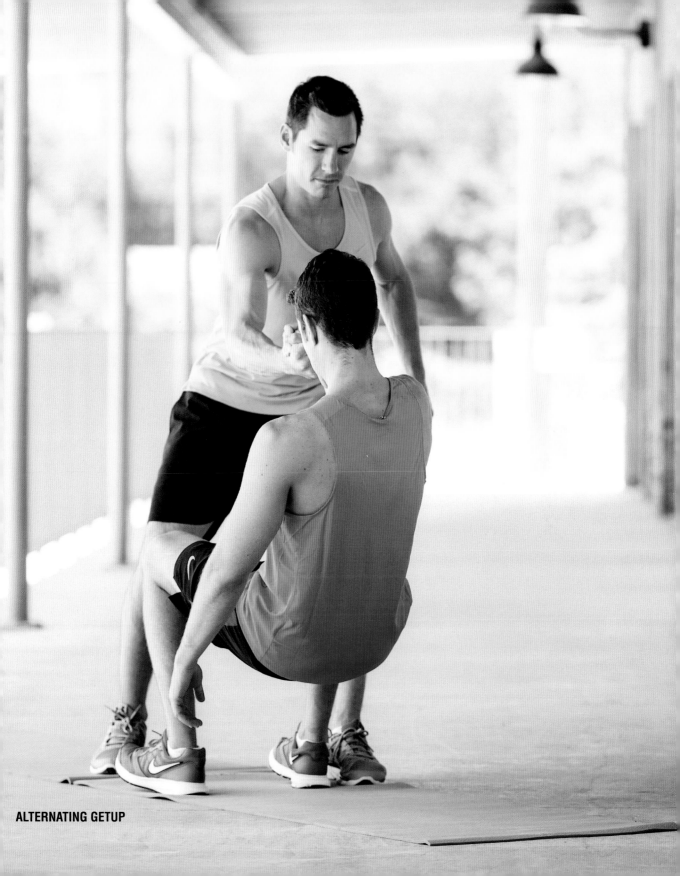

ALTERNATING GETUP

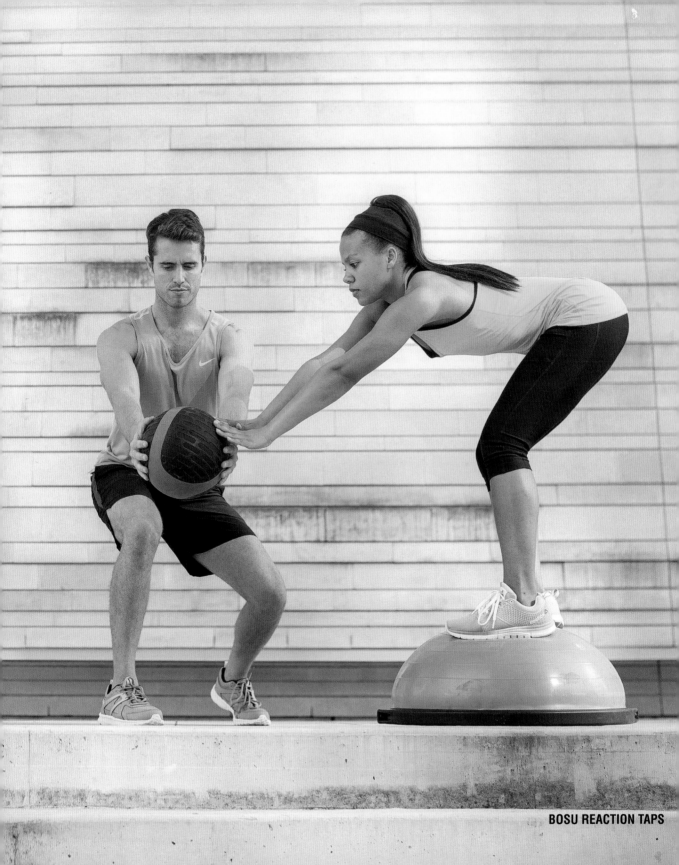

BOSU REACTION TAPS

TWISTED TABATA

This isn't a traditional Tabata (a HIIT variation). Focus on form, preparing for your heart rate to rise; 6 minutes might not seem long, but Tabatas are surprisingly tough.

YOU'LL NEED

Timer
Medicine ball
BOSU ball

CIRCUIT 1	EXERCISE	TIME	REST	PAGE
	Squat, Reach & Pass	30 secs	15 secs	50
	Sliding Chest Pass	30 secs	15 secs	54
	Perform 4 times total, resting 2 minutes after you finish all 4 rounds.			

CIRCUIT 2	EXERCISE	TIME	REST	PAGE
	Alternating Getup	30 secs	15 secs	102
	Coordinated Lunges	30 secs	15 secs	92
	Perform 4 times total, resting 2 minutes after you finish all 4 rounds.			

CIRCUIT 3	EXERCISE	TIME	REST	PAGE
	BOSU Reaction Taps	30 secs	15 secs	142
	BOSU Arm Wrestling	30 secs	15 secs	162
	Perform 4 times total, alternating roles after each round.			

LOWER-BODY BURNER

Focus on your bottom half— your glutes, quads, hamstrings, and calves—with this workout. Two rounds take just 15 minutes— perfect for lunchtime routines.

YOU'LL NEED

Timer
2 resistance bands

CIRCUIT	EXERCISE	TIME	REST	PAGE
	Reverse Lunge & Triceps Extension	50 secs	10 secs	42
	Side Lunge & Twist	50 secs	10 secs	38
	Leg Press	50 secs	10 secs	100
	Back-to-Back Squats	50 secs	10 secs	88
	Warrior III Leg Lifts (switching legs)	50 secs	10 secs	160
	V-Sit Adductor & Abductor	50 secs	10 secs	114
	Chair Pose on Toes	50 secs	60 secs	150
	Perform 2 times total, alternating roles after the first round.			

UPPER-BODY BURNER

This targets your back, chest, shoulders, biceps, and triceps. Because this routine takes only 15 minutes, consider combining it with another short workout.

YOU'LL NEED

Timer
Resistance band

	EXERCISE	TIME	REST	PAGE
CIRCUIT	Wheelbarrow Squat & Pushup	50 secs	10 secs	98
	Modified Pullup	50 secs	10 secs	106
	Resistance Band Chest Press & Row	50 secs	10 secs	48
	Superman Lats & Biceps Curls	50 secs	10 secs	40
	Resisted Shoulder Press	50 secs	10 secs	90
	Bridge Hold & Dip	50 secs	10 secs	112
	Standing Backbend	50 secs	60 secs	146

Perform 2 times total, alternating roles after each round.

CORE BLITZ

This is one of the shortest circuits in this book, and each exercise focuses on core strength, forcing you to work your abs, lower back, hips, and shoulder girdle.

YOU'LL NEED

Timer
Stability ball

	EXERCISE	TIME	REST	PAGE
CIRCUIT	Wheelbarrow Walk	50 secs	10 secs	96
	Stability Ball Situp & Pass	50 secs	10 secs	52
	Leg Throws	50 secs	10 secs	70
	Plank & Bridge	50 secs	10 secs	110
	Hand-Supported Double Boat Pose	50 secs	10 secs	148

Perform 2 times total, alternating roles after each round.

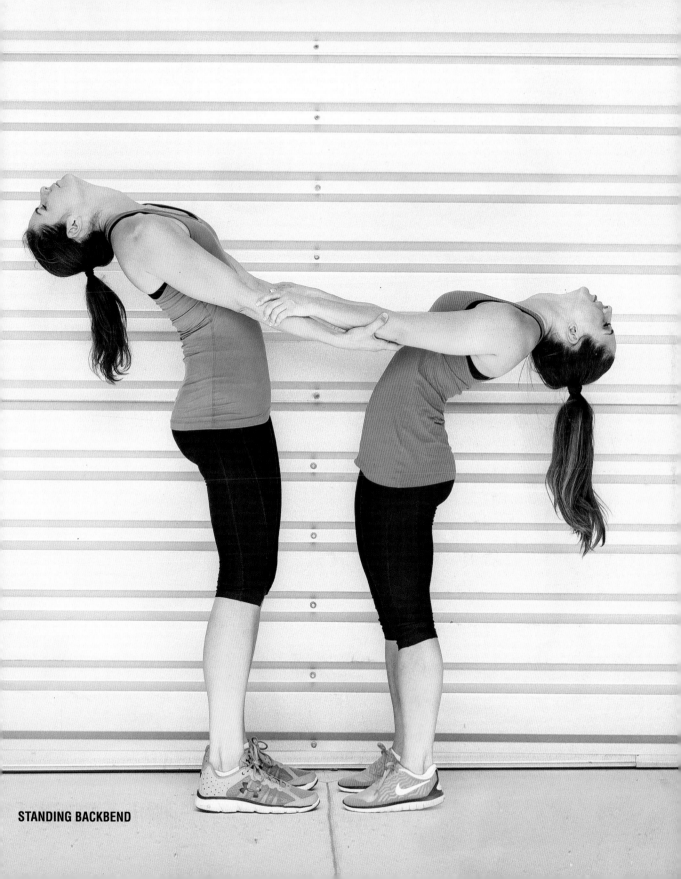

STANDING BACKBEND

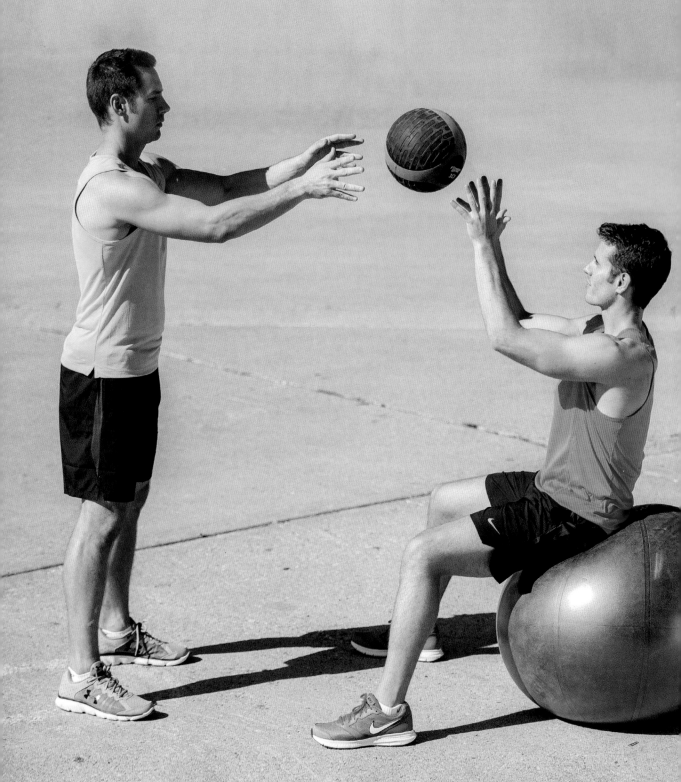

STABILITY BALL SITUP & MEDICINE BALL PASS

CELLULAR EXCITATION

You'll move constantly throughout this workout. Stay focused— mental and physical awareness are fundamental to maintaining proper form and putting in your best effort.

YOU'LL NEED

Timer
Resistance band
BOSU ball

	EXERCISE	TIME	REST	PAGE
CIRCUIT	Squat & Resistance Band Sprint	50 secs	10 secs	36
	Bear Crawl & Static Row	50 secs	10 secs	58
	BOSU Reaction Taps	50 secs	10 secs	142
	Alternating Getup	50 secs	10 secs	102
	Back-to-Back Squats	50 secs	10 secs	88
	Perform 4 times total, alternating roles after each round.			

COME ON STRONG

This workout incorporates almost as many intermediate-level moves as beginner moves. Each circuit will help you develop strength, power, agility, and endurance.

YOU'LL NEED

Timer   Dumbbell
Medicine ball   Stability ball

	EXERCISE	TIME	REST	PAGE
CIRCUIT 1	Squat, Reach & Pass	45 secs	15 secs	50
	Sliding Chest Pass	45 secs	15 secs	54
	Weighted Plank & Dumbbell Row	45 secs	15 secs	44
	Wall Squat & Overhead Dumbbell Shoulder Press	45 secs	15 secs	68
	Double Tree Pose	45 secs	60 secs	152
	Perform 2 times total, alternating roles after each round.			

	EXERCISE	TIME	REST	PAGE
CIRCUIT 2	Back-to-Back Squats	45 secs	15 secs	88
	Lateral Medicine Ball Toss	45 secs	15 secs	60
	Weighted Plank & Triceps Extension	45 secs	15 secs	46
	Wall Squat & Dip	45 secs	15 secs	94
	Double Dancer Pose	45 secs	60 secs	144
	Perform 2 times total, alternating roles after each round.			

	EXERCISE	TIME	REST	PAGE
CIRCUIT 3	Stability Ball Situp & Medicine Ball Pass	45 secs	15 secs	84
	Wall Squat & Medicine Ball Situp	45 secs	15 secs	64
	V-Sit Adductor & Abductor	45 secs	60 secs	114
	Perform 2 times total, alternating roles after each round.			

LEVEL 2 PROGRAM

The first two weeks of the Level 2 program incorporate four workouts and three days of rest, gradually ramping up the intensity to prepare you to tackle five workouts with two rest days the last two weeks of the program.

WEEK 1

DAY	WORKOUT	PAGE
1	Steady Cycle	199
2	Rest	
3	Power of 10 and Hard Core	200 and 204
4	Rest	
5	Steady Cycle	199
6	Hang in the Balance	200
7	Rest	

WEEK 2

DAY	WORKOUT	PAGE
1	The Countdown	198
2	Rest	
3	Power of 10 and Hard Core	200 and 204
4	Rest	
5	The Countdown	198
6	Hang in the Balance	200
7	Rest	

WEEK 3

DAY	WORKOUT	PAGE
1	The Countdown	198
2	The Push & Pull and Hard Core	206 and 204
3	Rest	
4	Perfect 10	202
5	The Push & Pull and Hard Core	206 and 204
6	The Heart Racer	203
7	Rest	

WEEK 4

DAY	WORKOUT	PAGE
1	The Spider	207
2	Butt Blaster and Hard Core	204
3	Rest	
4	The Spider	207
5	Butt Blaster and Hard Core	204
6	The Heart Racer	203
7	Rest	

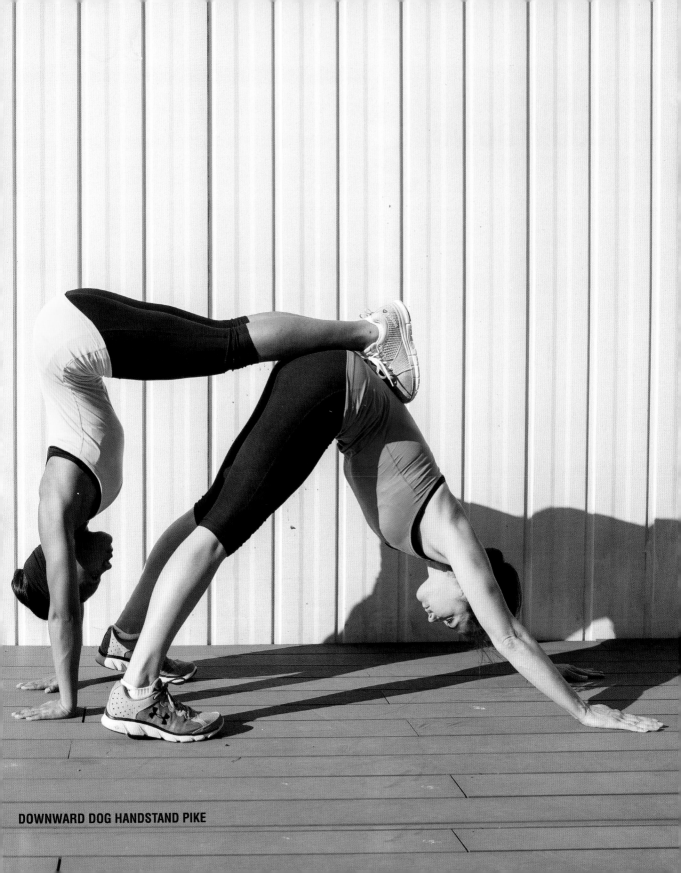

DOWNWARD DOG HANDSTAND PIKE

THE COUNTDOWN

What's different about this workout is the length of time you'll perform each exercise, going from 60 seconds to 45 seconds to 30 seconds.

YOU'LL NEED

Timer

Resistance band

BOSU ball

Medicine ball

CIRCUIT 1

EXERCISE	TIME	REST	PAGE
Sliding Chest Pass	60 secs		54
Squat, Reach & Pass	60 secs		50
Lateral Medicine Ball Toss	60 secs		60
BOSU Reaction Taps	60 secs		142
Alternating Getup	60 secs		102
King of the BOSU	60 secs		154
BOSU Arm Wrestling	60 secs		162

Perform 2 times total, alternating roles after the first round where appropriate and resting for 60 seconds only after completing both rounds.

CIRCUIT 2

EXERCISE	TIME	REST	PAGE
Sliding Chest Pass	45 secs		54
Squat, Reach & Pass	45 secs		50
Lateral Medicine Ball Toss	45 secs		60
BOSU Reaction Taps	45 secs		142
Alternating Getup	45 secs		102
King of the BOSU	45 secs		154
BOSU Arm Wrestling	45 secs		162

Perform 2 times total, alternating roles after the first round where appropriate and resting for 60 seconds only after completing both rounds.

CIRCUIT 3

EXERCISE	TIME	REST	PAGE
Sliding Chest Pass	30 secs		54
Squat, Reach & Pass	30 secs		50
Lateral Medicine Ball Toss	30 secs		60
BOSU Reaction Taps	30 secs		142
Alternating Getup	30 secs		102
King of the BOSU	30 secs		154
BOSU Arm Wrestling	30 secs		162

Perform 2 times total, alternating roles after the first round where appropriate and resting for 60 seconds only after completing both rounds.

STEADY CYCLE

If you keep the right pace, this strength-building circuit will take 41 minutes. Each circuit includes upper-body, lower-body, core, and balance training moves.

YOU'LL NEED

2 BOSU balls
2 resistance bands

2 medicine balls
Stability ball

CIRCUIT 1

EXERCISE	TIME	REST	PAGE
BOSU Squat & Resistance Band Row	50 secs	10 secs	66
Unstable Pushup & Medicine Ball Roll	50 secs	10 secs	62
Wall Squat & Dip	50 secs	10 secs	94
Plank & Bent-Over Row	50 secs	10 secs	108
Pedaling BOSU V-Sit	50 secs	10 secs	156

Perform 2 times total, alternating roles after the first round and resting for 60 seconds only after completing both rounds.

CIRCUIT 2

EXERCISE	TIME	REST	PAGE
Alternating Getup	50 secs	10 secs	102
Modified Pullup	50 secs	10 secs	106
Floating Plank & Shoulder Press	50 secs	10 secs	56
Leg Press	50 secs	10 secs	100
Pushing Side Planks	50 secs	10 secs	164

Perform 2 times total, alternating roles after the first round and resting for 60 seconds only after completing both rounds.

CIRCUIT 3

EXERCISE	TIME	REST	PAGE
BOSU Arm Wrestling	50 secs	10 secs	162
Wheelbarrow Squat & Pushup	50 secs	10 secs	98
Bridge Hold & Dip	50 secs	10 secs	112
V-Sit Adductor & Abductor	50 secs	10 secs	114
Wall Squat & Medicine Ball Situp	50 secs	10 secs	64

Perform 2 times total, alternating roles after the first round and resting for 60 seconds only after completing both rounds.

CIRCUIT 4

EXERCISE	TIME	REST	PAGE
King of the BOSU	50 secs	10 secs	154
Warrior III Leg Lifts (switching legs)	50 secs	10 secs	160
Stability Ball Plank	50 secs	10 secs	158
Leg Throws	50 secs	10 secs	70

Perform 2 times total, alternating roles after each round and resting for 60 seconds only after completing both rounds.

HANG IN THE BALANCE

This workout is guaranteed to deliver a few laughs as you and your partner cycle through stability-focused exercises designed to challenge and delight.

YOU'LL NEED

Timer
2 BOSU ball
2 resistance bands

2 stability balls
Medicine ball

CIRCUIT 1

EXERCISE	TIME	REST	PAGE
BOSU Squat & Resistance Band Row	50 secs	10 secs	66
Pedaling BOSU V-Sit	50 secs	10 secs	156
Stability Ball Plank	50 secs	10 secs	158
Chair Pose on Toes	60 secs		150

Perform 2 times total, resting for 60 seconds after completing both rounds.

CIRCUIT 2

EXERCISE	TIME	REST	PAGE
King of the BOSU	50 secs	10 secs	154
V-Sit Adductor & Abductor	50 secs	10 secs	114
Pushing Side Planks	50 secs	10 secs	164
Standing Backbend	60 secs		146

Perform 4 times total, alternating roles after each round and resting for 60 seconds after completing all the rounds.

CIRCUIT 3

EXERCISE	TIME	REST	PAGE
Single-Leg Stability Ball Battle	50 secs	10 secs	168
Warrior III Leg Lifts (switching legs)	50 secs	10 secs	160
Downward Dog Handstand Pike	50 secs	10 secs	166
Double Dancer Pose	60 secs		144

Perform 2 times total, alternating roles after the first round and resting for 60 secs after completing both rounds.

POWER OF 10

Don't let this short workout fool you—it's going to push your limits. The only breaks are between exercises and the time you'll use to regroup between each circuit.

YOU'LL NEED

Timer
Resistance band
2 medicine balls

CIRCUIT 1

EXERCISE	TIME	REST	PAGE
Bear Crawl & Static Row	20 secs	10 secs	58
Unstable Pushup & Medicine Ball Roll	20 secs	10 secs	62
Leg Throws	20 secs	10 secs	70

Perform 6 times total, alternating roles after each round and resting for 30 seconds after completing all the rounds.

CIRCUIT 2

EXERCISE	TIME	REST	PAGE
Wheelbarrow Walk	20 secs	10 secs	96
Wall Squat & Medicine Ball Situp	20 secs	10 secs	64
Floating Plank & Shoulder Press	20 secs	10 secs	56

Perform 6 times total, alternating roles after each round and resting for 30 seconds after completing all the rounds.

CIRCUIT 3

EXERCISE	TIME	REST	PAGE
Alternating Getup	20 secs	10 secs	102
Bridge Hold & Dip	20 secs	10 secs	112
Leg Press	20 secs	10 secs	100

Perform 6 times total, alternating roles after each round and resting for 30 seconds after completing all the rounds.

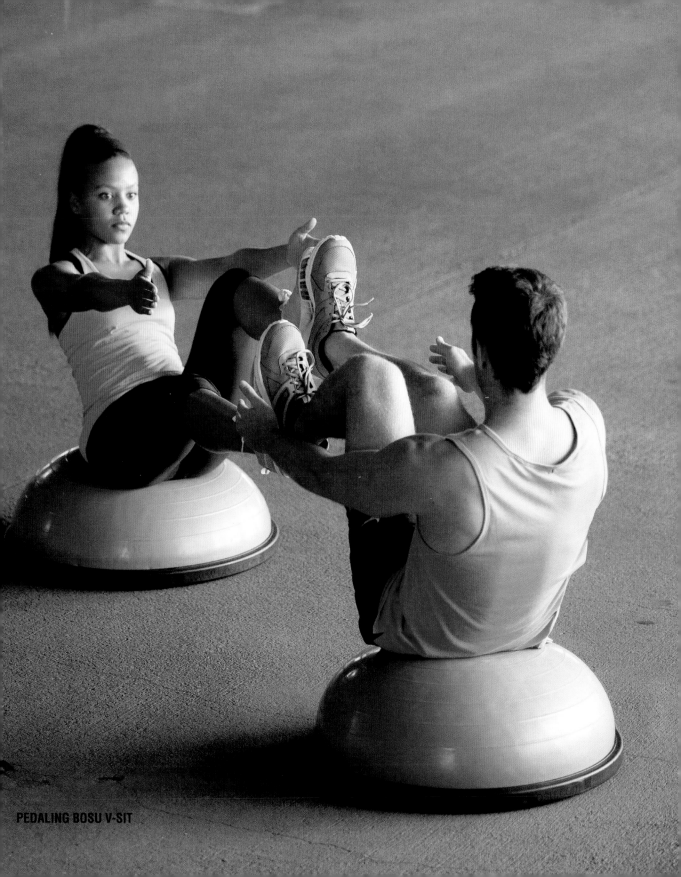

PEDALING BOSU V-SIT

LEVEL 2

PERFECT 10

This full-body workout might seem relatively easy, but looks can prove deceiving. You'll perform each circuit 20 times through—10 times per role before switching roles.

YOU'LL NEED

▶

No equipment needed

CIRCUIT 1

EXERCISE	REPS	REST	PAGE
Leg Press	10, 9, 8 …		100
Modified Pullup	10, 9, 8 …		106
Leg Throws	10, 9, 8 …		70

Perform without resting between exercises, counting down your reps per round—starting with 10 and ending with 1—before switching roles to repeat the entire circuit.

CIRCUIT 2

EXERCISE	REPS	REST	PAGE
Wheelbarrow Squat & Pushup	10, 9, 8 …		98
Plank & Bridge	10, 9, 8 …		110
Bridge Hold & Dip	10, 9, 8 …		112

Perform without resting between exercises, counting down your reps per round—starting with 10 and ending with 1—before switching roles to repeat the entire circuit.

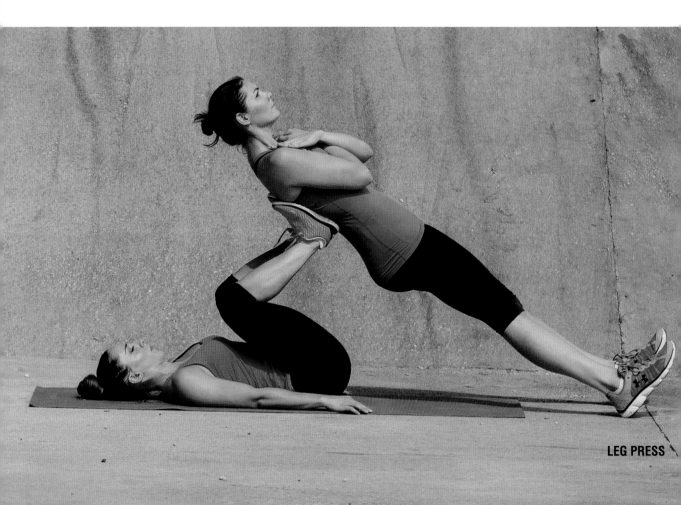

LEG PRESS

THE HEART RACER

It's time to get your heart rate up! This workout heavily focuses on cardiovascular moves, with brief rest periods to keep the intensity level high.

YOU'LL NEED

Resistance band	Medicine ball
2 BOSU balls	2 stability balls

CIRCUIT 1

EXERCISE	TIME	REST	PAGE
Bear Crawl & Static Row	50 secs	10 secs	58
Wheelbarrow Walk	50 secs	10 secs	96
Bear Crawl & Static Row	50 secs	10 secs	58
Wheelbarrow Walk	50 secs	10 secs	96

Perform 2 times total, alternating roles after each round.

CIRCUIT 2

EXERCISE	TIME	REST	PAGE
King of the BOSU	50 secs	10 secs	154
Alternating Getup	50 secs	10 secs	102
King of the BOSU	50 secs	10 secs	154
Alternating Getup	50 secs	10 secs	102

Perform 2 times total, alternating roles after each round.

CIRCUIT 3

EXERCISE	TIME	REST	PAGE
Single-Leg Stability Ball Battle (right leg)	50 secs	10 secs	168
Wheelbarrow Walk	50 secs	10 secs	96
Single-Leg Stability Ball Battle (left leg)	50 secs	10 secs	168
Wheelbarrow Walk	50 secs	10 secs	96

Perform 2 times total, alternating roles after each round.

CIRCUIT 4

EXERCISE	TIME	REST	PAGE
Wall Squat & Dip	50 secs	10 secs	94
Alternating Getup	50 secs	10 secs	102
Wall Squat & Dip	50 secs	10 secs	94
Alternating Getup	50 secs	10 secs	102

Perform 2 times total, alternating roles after each round.

CIRCUIT 5

EXERCISE	TIME	REST	PAGE
Coordinated Lunges	50 secs	10 secs	92
Lateral Medicine Ball Toss	50 secs	10 secs	60
Coordinated Lunges	50 secs	10 secs	92
Lateral Medicine Ball Toss	50 secs	10 secs	60

Perform 2 times total, alternating roles after each round.

CIRCUIT 6

EXERCISE	TIME	REST	PAGE
Unstable Pushup & Medicine Ball Roll	50 secs	10 secs	62
Pedaling BOSU V-Sit	50 secs	10 secs	156
Unstable Pushup & Medicine Ball Roll	50 secs	10 secs	62
Pedaling BOSU V-Sit	50 secs		156

Perform 2 times total, alternating roles after each round.

LEVEL 2

HARD CORE

This quick workout makes a perfect addition to a longer cardio routine or enables you to squeeze in exercises when you're short on time.

YOU'LL NEED

▶

Medicine ball
Stability ball

	EXERCISE	TIME	REST	PAGE
CIRCUIT	Sliding Chest Pass	60 secs		54
	Squat, Reach & Pass	60 secs		50
	Stability Ball Plank	60 secs		158
	Warrior III Leg Lifts (switching legs)	60 secs		160
	Pushing Side Planks	60 secs		164
	Downward Dog Handstand Pike	60 secs		166

Perform 4 times total, alternating roles after each round.

BUTT BLASTER

This routine alternates compound exercises that target multiple lower-body muscles and isolation exercises that focus on the glutes, hips, quads, and hamstrings.

YOU'LL NEED

▶

Timer
2 resistance bands

	EXERCISE	TIME	REST	PAGE
CIRCUIT 1	Wall Squat & Dip	45 secs	15 secs	94
	Leg Press	45 secs	15 secs	100
	Coordinated Hamstring Curls	45 secs	15 secs	78
	Warrior III Leg Lifts (switching legs)	45 secs	15 secs	160

Perform 4 times total, alternating roles after each round and resting for 2 minutes after completing each round.

	EXERCISE	TIME	REST	PAGE
CIRCUIT 2	Wall Squat & Medicine Ball Situp	45 secs	15 secs	64
	BOSU Squat & Resistance Band Row	45 secs	15 secs	66
	Wall Squat & Bulgarian Split Squat	45 secs	15 secs	118
	Plank & Bridge	45 secs	15 secs	110

Perform 4 times total, alternating roles after each round and resting for 2 minutes after completing each round.

	EXERCISE	TIME	REST	PAGE
CIRCUIT 3	Wall Squat & Overhead Dumbbell Shoulder Press	45 secs	15 secs	68
	Assisted Pistol Squat	45 secs	15 secs	116
	V-Sit Adductor & Abductor	45 secs	15 secs	114
	Bridge Hold & Dip	45 secs	15 secs	112

Perform 4 times total, alternating roles after each round.

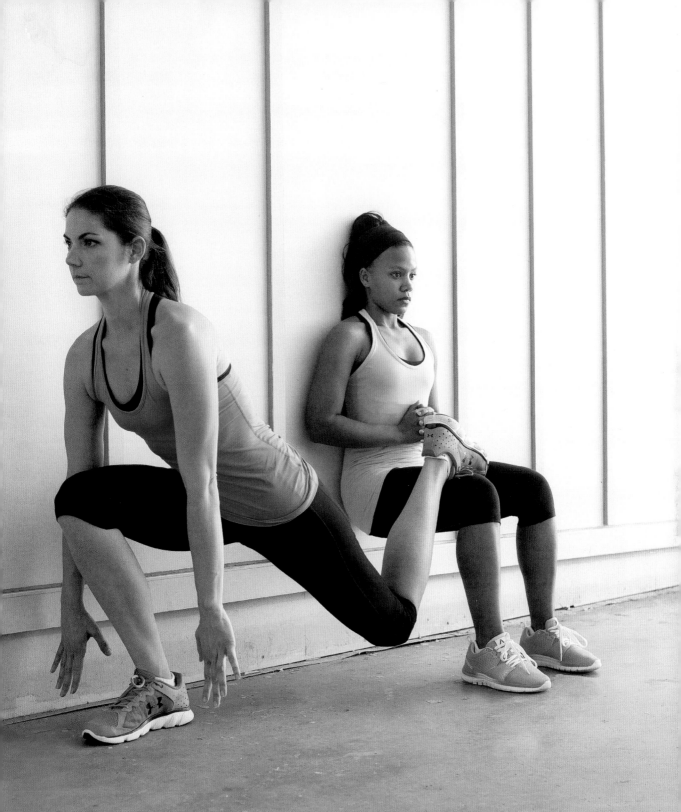

WALL SQUAT & SPLIT SQUAT

LEVEL 2

THE PUSH & PULL

This upper-body routine incorporates pushing moves for your chest, shoulders, and triceps as well as pulling moves for your back and biceps.

YOU'LL NEED

- Resistance band
- 2 BOSU balls
- 2 medicine balls
- 2 dumbbells

CIRCUIT 1

EXERCISE	TIME	REST	PAGE
Bear Crawl & Static Row	50 secs	10 secs	58
Twisting Squat & BOSU Pushup	50 secs	10 secs	122
Unstable Pushup & Medicine Ball Roll	50 secs	10 secs	62
Floating Plank & Shoulder Press	50 secs	10 secs	56

Perform 2 times total, alternating roles after the first round.

CIRCUIT 2

EXERCISE	TIME	REST	PAGE
BOSU Arm Wrestling	50 secs	10 sec	162
Modified Pullup	50 secs	10 secs	106
Elevated Pushup & Chest Press	50 secs	10 secs	128
Wall Squat & Overhead Dumbbell Shoulder Press	50 secs	10 secs	68

Perform 2 times total, alternating roles after the first round.

CIRCUIT 3

EXERCISE	TIME	REST	PAGE
Alternating Getup	50 secs	10 secs	102
Wheelbarrow Squat & Pushup	50 secs	10 secs	98
Plank & Bent-Over Row	50 secs	10 secs	108
Handstand Shoulder Press	50 secs	10 secs	126

Perform 2 times total, alternating roles after the first round.

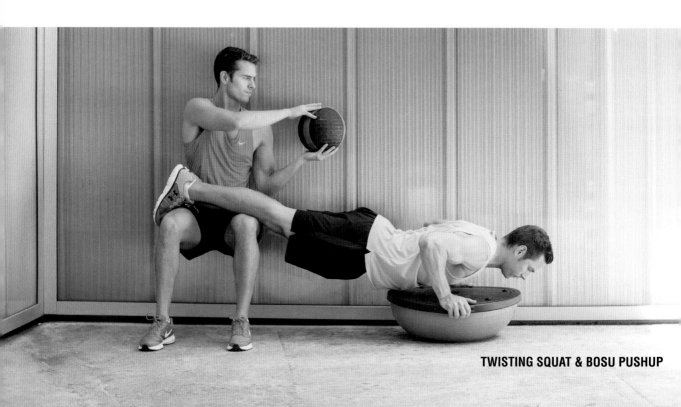

TWISTING SQUAT & BOSU PUSHUP

THE SPIDER

Spiders have eight legs, and this workout does things in eights, leading to its name. You'll perform eight exercises eight times for eight reps each—and quickly.

YOU'LL NEED

Dumbbell
Medicine ball

CIRCUIT 1

EXERCISE	REPS	REST	PAGE
Wheelbarrow Squat & Pushup	8		98

Perform 8 times total, alternating roles after completing your reps and resting for 30 seconds only after completing all 8 rounds.

CIRCUIT 2

EXERCISE	REPS	REST	PAGE
Weighted Plank & Lateral Hops	8		134

Perform 8 times total, alternating roles after completing your reps and resting for 30 seconds only after completing all 8 rounds.

CIRCUIT 3

EXERCISE	REPS	REST	PAGE
Weighted Plank & Dumbbell Row	8 per arm		44

Perform 8 times total, alternating roles after completing your reps and resting for 30 seconds only after completing all 8 rounds.

CIRCUIT 4

EXERCISE	REPS	REST	PAGE
Wall Squat & Medicine Ball Situp	8		64

Perform 8 times total, alternating roles after completing your reps and resting for 30 seconds only after completing all 8 rounds.

CIRCUIT 5

EXERCISE	REPS	REST	PAGE
Wall Squat & Dip	8		94

Perform 8 times total, alternating roles after completing your reps and resting for 30 seconds only after completing all 8 rounds.

CIRCUIT 6

EXERCISE	REPS	REST	PAGE
Leg Press	8		100

Perform 8 times total, alternating roles after completing your reps and resting for 30 seconds only after completing all 8 rounds.

CIRCUIT 7

EXERCISE	REPS	REST	PAGE
Modified Pullup	8		106

Perform 8 times total, alternating roles after completing your reps and resting for 30 seconds only after completing all 8 rounds.

CIRCUIT 8

EXERCISE	REPS	REST	PAGE
Leg Throws	8		70

Perform 8 times total, alternating roles after completing your reps.

LEVEL 3 PROGRAM

This intense program isn't for newbies—the exercises, workouts, and program progression are for individuals with advanced skills and fitness abilities.
Omit at least one workout per week if you're not completely ready for Level 3.

WEEK 1

DAY	WORKOUT	PAGE
1	Next-Level HIIT	210
2	Balancing Act	211
3	Rest	
4	Guns & Buns Countdown	213
5	Balancing Act	211
6	Next-Level HIIT	210
7	Rest	

WEEK 2

DAY	WORKOUT	PAGE
1	Chest & Abs and Quick & Dirty	214 and 213
2	45-Minute Pyramid	215
3	Rest	
4	Toasted	215
5	Chest & Abs	214
6	Toasted	215
7	Rest	

WEEK 3

DAY	WORKOUT	PAGE
1	Chest & Abs and Quick & Dirty	214 and 213
2	45-Minute Pyramid	215
3	Rest	
4	Tabata Master Class	216
5	Sweat Social	210
6	Chest & Abs	214
7	Toasted	215

WEEK 4

DAY	WORKOUT	PAGE
1	Balancing Act	211
2	The Crucible	218
3	Rest	
4	Tabata Master Class	216
5	Sweat Social	210
6	Toasted	215
7	Chest & Abs	214

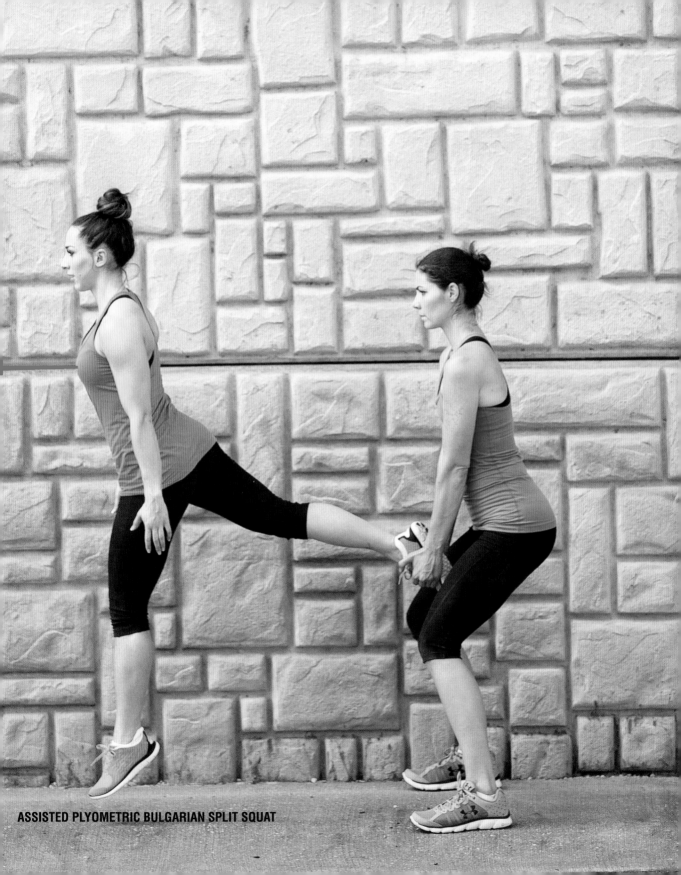

ASSISTED PLYOMETRIC BULGARIAN SPLIT SQUAT

NEXT-LEVEL HIIT

This workout uses HIIT—but it amps everything up. Each circuit includes an upper-body, lower-body, core, and cardiovascular challenge for a total-body routine.

YOU'LL NEED

Stability ball   Medicine ball
BOSU ball

CIRCUIT 1

EXERCISE	TIME	REST	PAGE
Weighted Plank & Lateral Hops	20 secs	10 secs	134
Coordinated Stability Ball Lunges (switch legs every round)	20 secs	10 secs	80
Power Plank & Chest Press	20 secs	10 secs	72
Stability Ball Situp & Medicine Ball Pass	20 secs	10 secs	84

Perform 8 times total, alternating roles after each round.

CIRCUIT 2

EXERCISE	TIME	REST	PAGE
Fireman's Carry	40 secs	20 secs	138
Wall Squat & Bulgarian Split Squat (switch legs every round)	40 secs	20 secs	118
Elevated Pushup & Chest Press	40 secs	20 secs	128
Side Plank & Hip Adduction (switch legs every round)	40 secs	20 secs	170

Perform 4 times total, alternating roles after each round.

CIRCUIT 3

EXERCISE	TIME	REST	PAGE
BOSU Ball Battle	30 secs	10 secs	180
Assisted Pistol Squat (switch legs every round)	30 secs	10 secs	116
Plank & Bent-Over Row	30 secs	10 secs	108
Stability Ball Balance & Jab	30 secs	10 secs	176

Perform 4 times total, alternating roles after each round.

SWEAT SOCIAL

This workout is designed to tax your cardiovascular system. While it includes exercises from Level 1 and Level 2, don't assume it'll be remotely easy.

YOU'LL NEED

Resistance band   Stability ball
Medicine ball   BOSU ball

CIRCUIT

EXERCISE	TIME	REST	PAGE
Fireman's Carry	60 secs		138
Squat & Resistance Band Sprint	60 secs		36
Sliding Chest Pass	60 secs		54
Bear Crawl & Static Row	60 secs		58
Wheelbarrow Walk	60 secs		96
Alternating Getups	60 secs		102
Weighted Plank & Lateral Hops	60 secs		134
Assisted Pistol Squat (switch legs every round)	60 secs		116
Power Plank & Chest Press	30 secs	30 secs	72

Perform 4 times total, alternating roles after each round.

BALANCING ACT

This progressive balance-focused workout combines cardio, strength, and stability exercises that will fire up your core, specifically your abs, lower back, hips, and shoulders.

YOU'LL NEED

Stability ball
Medicine ball
BOSU ball

	EXERCISE	TIME	REST	PAGE
CIRCUIT	Kneeling Balance & Pass	45 secs		174
	Double Bridge	30 secs	15 secs	132
	Stability Ball Balance & Jab	45 secs		176
	Downward Dog Handstand Pike	30 secs	15 secs	166
	BOSU Pushup & Shoulder Squat	45 secs		74
	Standing Backbend	30 secs	15 secs	146
	Coordinated Stability Ball Lunges	45 secs		80
	Stacked Plank	30 secs	15 secs	172
	Stability Ball Reverse Curl & Triceps Rollout	45 secs		76
	Flying Bird Pose	30 secs	15 secs	178
	Coordinated Stability Ball Hamstring Curls	45 secs		78
	Double Dancer Pose	30 secs	60 secs	144

Perform 2 times total, alternating roles after each round.

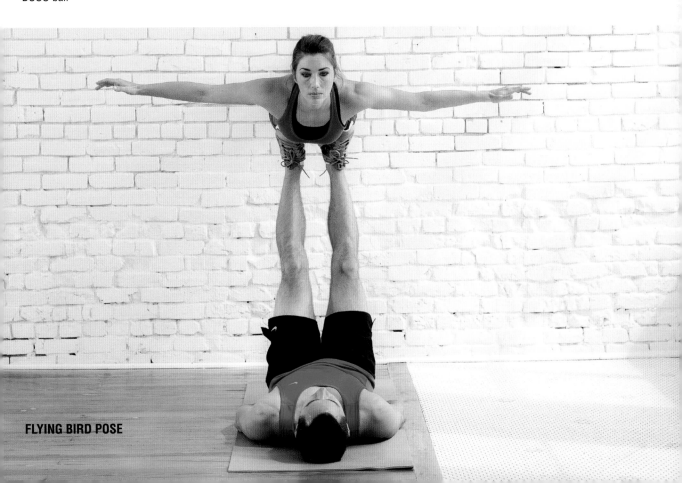

FLYING BIRD POSE

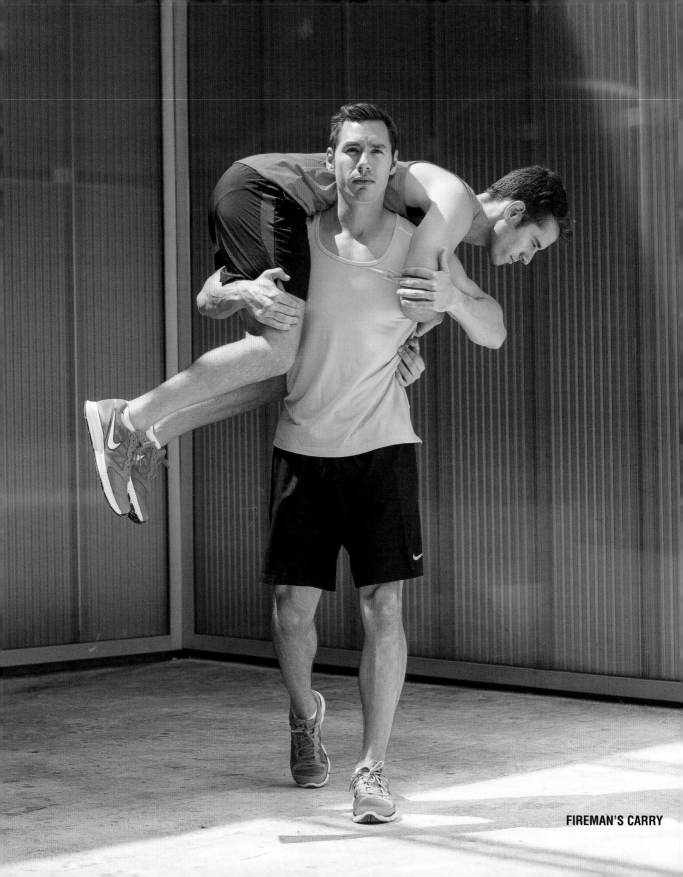

FIREMAN'S CARRY

QUICK & DIRTY

	EXERCISE	TIME	REST	PAGE
CIRCUIT	Fireman's Carry	60 secs		138
	Linked-Leg Pushups	60 secs		136
	Situp to Square Pike	30 secs		124
	Perform 4 times total, alternating roles after each round.			

This is the shortest Level 3 workout. Because you don't rest, your heart rate will soar. Pair this workout with another Level 3 workout for an extra challenge.

YOU'LL NEED

No equipment needed

GUNS & BUNS COUNTDOWN

	EXERCISE	REPS	REST	PAGE
CIRCUIT	BOSU Pushup & Shoulder Squat	15, 14 …		74
	Bridge Hold & Dip	15, 14 …		112
	Wall Squat & Overhead Dumbbell Shoulder Press	15, 14 …		68
	Perform 15 times total, reducing the number of reps each round—starting at 15 and going to 1— and alternating roles after each round.			

Each exercise in this workout combines an upper-body and a lower-body move. You'll start with the greatest number of reps and work your way down.

YOU'LL NEED

BOSU ball
2 dumbbells

LEVEL 3

CHEST & ABS

This focuses on your chest and abs—with a little supplemental upper-body work thrown in. If you want an extra burn, pair this with the Quick & Dirty workout.

YOU'LL NEED

BOSU ball
Stability ball
2 dumbbells

Medicine ball
Timer

CIRCUIT 1

EXERCISE	REPS	REST	PAGE
Power Plank & Chest Press	8.6		72
Stability Ball Reverse Curl & Triceps Rollout	8.6		76
Situp to Square Pike	8.6		124

Perform 4 times total, alternating roles after each round where appropriate. For rounds 1 and 2, perform 8 reps. For rounds 3 and 4, perform 6 reps. Rest 60 seconds after completing all the rounds.

CIRCUIT 2

EXERCISE	TIME	REST	PAGE
Single-Leg Stability Ball Battle	45 secs	15 secs	168
Weighted Plank & Dumbbell Chest Press	45 secs	15 secs	82
Stability Ball Situp & Medicine Ball Pass	45 secs	15 secs	84

Perform 6 times total, alternating roles after each round and resting 60 seconds after completing all the rounds.

CIRCUIT 3

EXERCISE	TIME	REST	PAGE
Elevated Pushup & Chest Press	40 secs	20 secs	128
Modified Pullup	40 secs	20 secs	106
Handstand Shoulder Press	40 secs	20 secs	126

Perform 6 times total, alternating roles after each round and resting 60 seconds after completing all the rounds.

CIRCUIT 4

EXERCISE	TIME	REST	PAGE
Linked-Leg Pushups	30 secs		136
Flying Bird Pose	60 secs		178

Perform 4 times total, alternating roles after each round.

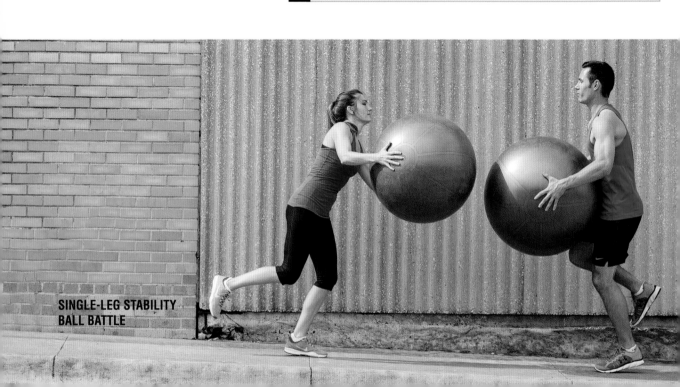

SINGLE-LEG STABILITY BALL BATTLE

TOASTED

Toasted is exactly what your lower body will feel like after this killer leg routine. Each circuit taxes the major leg muscles—and the burn builds with moves that target your core.

YOU'LL NEED

Stability ball   Timer

CIRCUIT 1	EXERCISE	TIME	REST	PAGE
	Coordinated Lunges	60 secs		92
	Wall Squat & Bulgarian Split Squat	60 secs		118
	Kneeling Hamstring Curls	30 secs		120
	Side Plank & Hip Adduction	30 secs		170

Perform 4 times total, alternating roles and legs (as needed) after each round, and rest for 2 minutes after all the rounds.

CIRCUIT 2	EXERCISE	TIME	REST	PAGE
	Fireman's Carry	60 secs		138
	Assisted Pistol Squat	45 secs		116
	Coordinated Stability Ball Hamstring Curls	45 secs		78
	Warrior III Leg Lifts	30 secs		160

Perform 4 times total, alternating roles and legs (as needed) after each round, and rest for 2 minutes after all the rounds.

CIRCUIT 3	EXERCISE	TIME	REST	PAGE
	Weighted Plank & Lateral Hops	90 secs		134
	Coordinated Stability Ball Lunges	60 secs		80
	Assisted Plyometric Bulgarian Split Squat	30 secs		130
	Double Bridge	30 secs		132

Perform 4 times total, alternating roles and legs (as needed) after each round.

45-MINUTE PYRAMID

After performing a full pyramid (going from a high rep number to a lower one), you'll switch roles. Your goal is to complete as many pyramids as you can in 45 minutes.

YOU'LL NEED

2 dumbbells   Medicine ball

CIRCUIT	EXERCISE	REPS	REST	PAGE
	Weighted Plank & Dumbbell Chest Press	30		82
	Stability Ball Situp & Medicine Ball Pass	25		84
	Assisted Plyometric Bulgarian Split Squat	10 per leg		130
	Twisting Squat & BOSU Pushup	15		122
	Modified Pullup	12		106
	Handstand Shoulder Press	10		126
	Kneeling Hamstring Curls	8		120
	Stability Ball Reverse Curl & Triceps Rollout	5		76

Perform the designated reps for each exercise without resting between sets, switching roles after completing one round. Perform the circuit again, and continue to switch roles after each full round, counting how many pyramids you complete in 45 minutes.

LEVEL 3

TABATA MASTER CLASS

You'll blast calories and keep your metabolic fire burning for hours after this 35-minute HIIT variation workout. Stick with each exercise for an entire circuit.

YOU'LL NEED

Stability ball
2 BOSU balls
Medicine ball

CIRCUIT 1

EXERCISE	TIME	REST	PAGE
Alternating Getup	20 secs	10 secs	102
Assisted Plyometric Bulgarian Split Squat	20 secs	10 secs	130
Perform 4 times total without switching roles.			

CIRCUIT 2

EXERCISE	TIME	REST	PAGE
Alternating Getup	20 secs	10 secs	102
Assisted Plyometric Bulgarian Split Squat	20 secs	10 secs	130
Switch roles from Tabata 1. Perform 4 times total.			

CIRCUIT 3

EXERCISE	TIME	REST	PAGE
Stability Ball Balance & Jab	20 secs	10 secs	176
Linked-Leg Pushups	20 secs	10 secs	136
Perform 4 times total without switching roles.			

CIRCUIT 4

EXERCISE	TIME	REST	PAGE
Stability Ball Balance & Jab	20 secs	10 secs	176
Linked-Leg Pushups	20 secs	10 secs	136
Switch roles from Tabata 3. Perform 4 times total.			

CIRCUIT 5

EXERCISE	TIME	REST	PAGE
Kneeling Balance & Pass	20 secs	10 secs	174
Situp to Square Pike	20 secs	10 secs	124
Perform 4 times total without switching roles.			

CIRCUIT 6

EXERCISE	TIME	REST	PAGE
Kneeling Balance & Pass	20 secs	10 secs	174
Situp to Square Pike	20 secs	10 secs	124
Switch roles from Tabata 5. Perform 4 times total.			

CIRCUIT 7

EXERCISE	TIME	REST	PAGE
BOSU Arm Wrestling	20 secs	10 secs	162
Weighted Plank & Lateral Hops	20 secs	10 secs	134
Perform 4 times total without switching roles.			

CIRCUIT 8

EXERCISE	TIME	REST	PAGE
BOSU Arm Wrestling	20 secs	10 secs	162
Weighted Plank & Lateral Hops	20 secs	10 secs	134
Switch roles from Tabata 7. Perform 4 times total.			

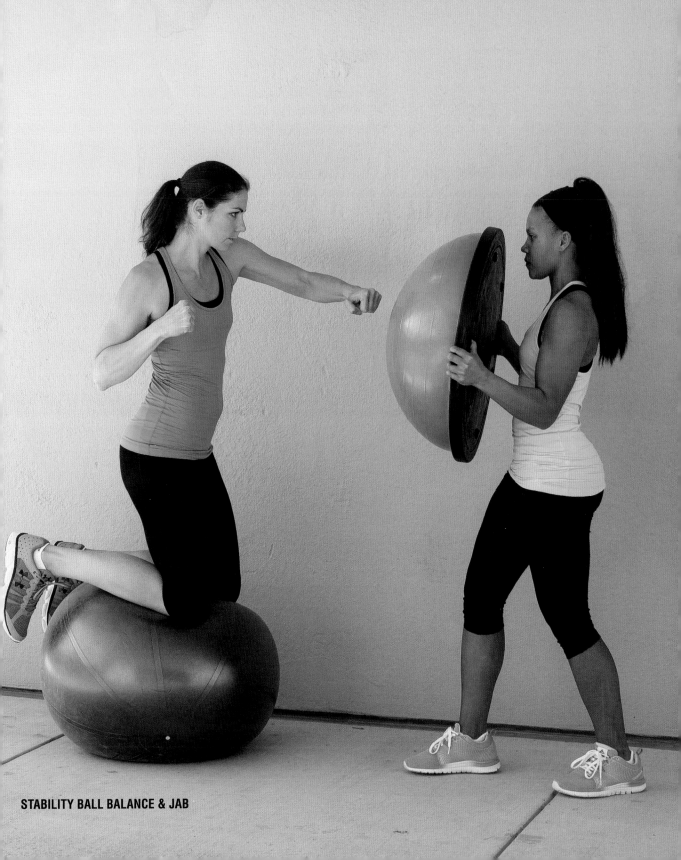

STABILITY BALL BALANCE & JAB

LEVEL 3

THE CRUCIBLE

This workout is what you've been working toward—the ultimate routine that lasts a full 79 minutes. This will test your mettle while targeting all major muscle groups.

YOU'LL NEED

Stability ball

CIRCUIT 1

EXERCISE	TIME	REST	PAGE
Fireman's Carry	2 mins	30 secs	138
Weighted Plank & Lateral Hops	60 secs	30 secs	134
Modified Pullup	50 secs	10 secs	106
Linked-Leg Pushups	50 secs	10 secs	136
Modified Pullup	50 secs	10 secs	106
Linked-Leg Pushups	50 secs	10 secs	136
Handstand Shoulder Press	50 secs	10 secs	126
Wall Squat & Dip	50 secs	10 secs	94
Handstand Shoulder Press	50 secs	10 secs	126
Wall Squat & Dip	50 secs	10 secs	94

Perform 2 times total, alternating roles after each round and resting for 2 minutes after completing both rounds.

CIRCUIT 2

EXERCISE	TIME	REST	PAGE
Fireman's Carry	2 mins	30 secs	138
Weighted Plank & Lateral Hops	60 secs	30 secs	134
Assisted Pistol Squat	50 secs	10 secs	116
Double Bridge	50 secs	10 secs	132
Assisted Pistol Squat (opposite leg)	50 secs	10 secs	116
Double Bridge	50 secs	10 secs	132
Assisted Plyometric Bulgarian Split Squat	50 secs	10 secs	130
Leg Press	50 secs	10 secs	100
Assisted Plyometric Bulgarian Split Squat (opposite leg)	50 secs	10 secs	130
Leg Press	50 secs	10 secs	100

Perform 2 times total, alternating roles after each round and resting for 2 minutes after completing both rounds.

CIRCUIT 3

EXERCISE	TIME	REST	PAGE
Fireman's Carry	2 mins	30 secs	138
Weighted Plank & Lateral Hops	60 secs	30 secs	134
Wheelbarrow Walk	50 secs	10 secs	96
Coordinated Stability Ball Hamstring Curls	50 secs	10 secs	78
Wheelbarrow Walk	50 secs	10 secs	96
Coordinated Stability Ball Hamstring Curls	50 secs	10 secs	78
Situp to Square Pike	50 secs	10 secs	124
Leg Throws	50 secs	10 secs	70
Situp to Square Pike	50 secs	10 secs	124
Leg Throws	50 secs	10 secs	70
Side Plank & Hip Adduction	50 secs	10 secs	170

Perform 2 times total, alternating roles after each round and resting for 2 minutes after completing both rounds.

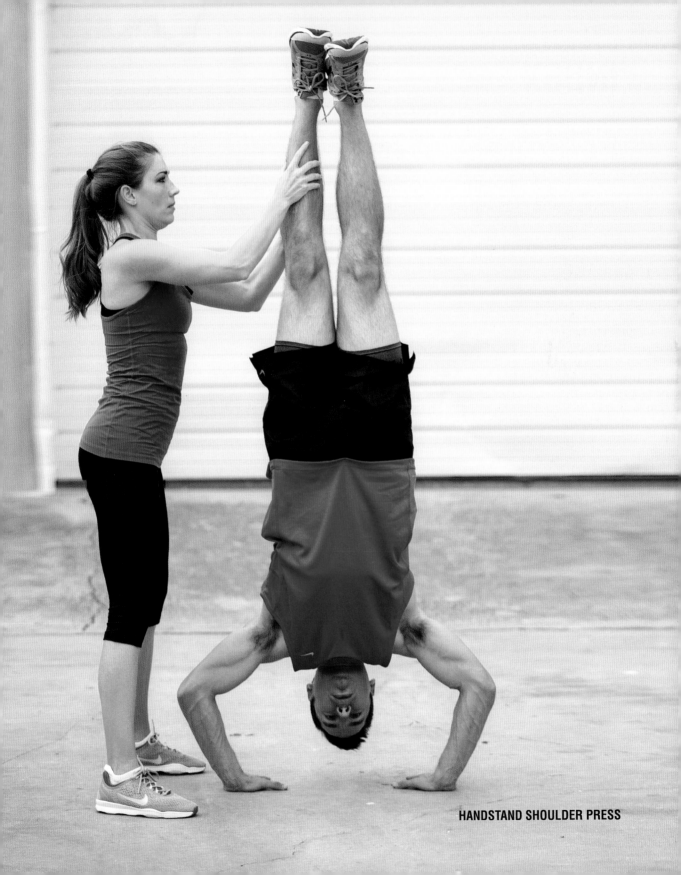

HANDSTAND SHOULDER PRESS

INDEX

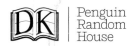

Publisher: Mike Sanders
Associate Publisher: Billy Fields
Acquisitions Editor: Nathalie Mornu
Development Editor: Christopher Stolle
Cover Designer: Harriet Yeomans
Book Designer: Mandy Earey
Art Director: Nigel Wright
Photographer: Dennis Burnett
Prepress Technician: Brian Massey
Proofreader: Laura Caddell
Indexer: Heather McNeill

First American Edition, 2016
Published in the United States by DK Publishing
6081 E. 82nd Street, Indianapolis, Indiana 46250

Copyright © 2016 Dorling Kindersley Limited
A Penguin Random House Company
16 17 18 19   10 9 8 7 6 5 4 3 2 1
001–295073–December/2016

Published in the United States by Dorling Kindersley Limited.

ISBN: 978-1-46545-348-8
Library of Congress Catalog Card Number: 2016941028

Note: This publication contains the opinions and ideas of its author(s).
It is intended to provide helpful and informative material on the subject
matter covered. It is sold with the understanding that the author(s) and publisher
are not engaged in rendering professional services in the book. If the reader
requires personal assistance or advice, a competent professional should be
consulted. The author(s) and publisher specifically disclaim any responsibility
for any liability, loss, or risk, personal or otherwise, which is incurred as a
consequence, directly or indirectly, of the use and application of any of the
contents of this book.

Trademarks: All terms mentioned in this book that are known to be or
are suspected of being trademarks or service marks have been appropriately
capitalized. Alpha Books, DK, and Penguin Random House LLC cannot attest
to the accuracy of this information. Use of a term in this book should not
be regarded as affecting the validity of any trademark or service mark.

DK books are available at special discounts when purchased in bulk for sales
promotions, premiums, fund-raising, or educational use. For details, contact:
DK Publishing Special Markets, 345 Hudson Street, New York,
New York 10014 or SpecialSales@dk.com.

Printed and bound in China

All images © Dorling Kindersley Limited

For further information see: www.dkimages.com

www.dk.com

A WORLD OF IDEAS:
SEE ALL THERE IS TO KNOW

About the Author

Laura Williams, MSEd, ACSM EP-C, has a master's degree in
exercise and sport science from the University of Mary Hardin–Baylor
and is a certified exercise physiologist through the American College
of Sports Medicine. She writes for Thrillist, Verywell, SheKnows, and
Onnit, and she's been featured in *Shape*, *The Huffington Post*,
Cosmopolitan, and *Real Simple*. Laura also runs her own healthy
living website: Girls Gone Sporty (girlsgonesporty.com).

Acknowledgments

A huge thanks is due to everyone at DK Books for this opportunity as
well as the fabulous group of individuals who worked tirelessly behind
the scenes to make this book happen. A special thank you goes out to
Nathalie Mornu and Christopher Stolle for their constant willingness
to answer questions and offer great insight throughout this process.

Thank you to Dennis Burnett for his photographs and to the models for
their long hours of hard work and their good humor while learning and
demonstrating the partner exercises. And a special thank you to Nigel
Wright's art direction before, during, and after the photo shoot. Your keen
eye for detail and your perfectionism are what take this book to the next
level. Without all of you, this book wouldn't be the masterpiece it is.

Well-deserved thanks also go to Catherine Connelly, Anthony Schneck,
and Rachel Berman—you've all been incredibly understanding, flexible,
and supportive, and the cumulative opportunities you've provided are
what made this book possible. I'd like to thank Dr. Colin Wilborn and
Dr. Cliffa Foster from the University of Mary Hardin–Baylor for lighting
a spark in me and supporting my continued education, even when it
wasn't easy. Your belief in me means more than you'll ever know.

To Kacie O'Kelley, Amy Loomis, Rebekah Meeks, Buffy McDaniel,
and Sara Parker—near or far, close or apart, whether we talk daily
or almost never at all, I can't imagine my life without friendships. You're
the definition of strong, powerful women whose kindness, courage, and
humor inspire me to keep on keepin' on, no matter the adversity. These
sentiments also apply to my sisters, Mary McCoy and Tanya Farman.

To my wonderful family—parents, in-laws, siblings, sisters- and
brothers-in-laws, and nieces—you're what make my heart tick. Know that
each of you—Greg and Geri; Ron and Gail; David and Tanya; Juliana and
Alexandra; Mary, Gabby, and Danny; Jeff and Julie; Kaitlyn and Cassie;
Adam; and Ben—have forever shaped who I am.

Finally—and most importantly—to my amazing husband, Lance: thank
you. Thank you for putting up with me when I decided to quit my job and
pursue writing. Thank you for supporting me through crazy deadlines and
stressful paychecks. Thank you for believing in me and encouraging me,
especially when I struggled to believe in and encourage myself. It's been
an awesome 13 years—I'm looking forward to many, many more.

Publisher's Acknowledgments

The publisher would like to thank Joey Kelly, Shannon Nicole Kerlin,
Bryanna Moody, Meredy Russell, Brad Snedden, and Laura Williams for
their time and effort in learning and executing the exercises in this book.